INFERTILITY

SECOND EDITION

Infertility
A Guide for the Childless Couple

Barbara Eck Menning, R.N., M.P.H.

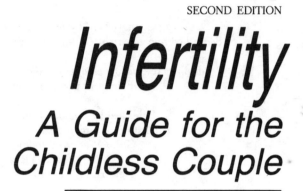

Prentice Hall Press

New York   London   Toronto   Sydney   Tokyo

Published by Prentice Hall Press
A Division of Simon & Schuster, Inc.
Gulf + Western Building
One Gulf + Western Plaza
New York, NY   10023

This is a second edition of a book originally published in 1977 by Prentice-Hall, Inc.

PRENTICE HALL PRESS is a registered trademark of Simon & Schuster, Inc.

Library of Congress Cataloging-in-Publication Data

Menning, Barbara Eck.
Infertility: a guide for the childless couple.

Bibliography: p.
Includes index.
1. Infertility.   2. Childlessness.   3. Infertility—
Psychological aspects.   I. Title.
RC889.M38   1988   618.1′78   87-19343
ISBN 0-13-464330-5

Manufactured in the United States of America

10   9   8   7   6   5   4   3

To those who are infertile
and to those who have been infertile,
this book is dedicated.

Acknowledgments

There are, of course, many people to thank. Writing a book is not easy, and revising one may even be harder. It certainly is not a solo performance. First and foremost, I must thank my children, Matthew, Jonathan, and Rebecca, for their patience and support. The first book was hammered out on an old Smith-Corona typewriter; this revision, appropriately, was rendered on a state-of-the-art word processor.

My most sincere appreciation for reading and advising me on the medical aspects of the book goes to Dr. Isaac Schiff of the Fertility, Endocrine, and Menopause Unit of the Brigham and Women's Hospital in Boston. Not only has Isaac been a good personal friend for many years, he has also served RESOLVE, Inc., in numerous capacities, including as a board member and a medical advisor.

Many thanks also go to Diane Clapp, R.N., a counselor and writer on the staff of RESOLVE for many years, who served as my research assistant in the revision project. She helped gather timely articles and readings so I was able to work "long distance" from Cape Cod, and she suggested the areas that needed changing. Diane and I go way back to the "kitchen table" days of RESOLVE, and I value our friendship as I value her great loyalty to RESOLVE and her important writing, public speaking, and work in the area of infertility.

Finally, I want to thank Bev Freeman, current executive director of RESOLVE, for her support and encouragement of this revision. She and her staff gave me unrestricted access to their library and materials and were available to answer questions whenever I needed them. Two former staff members of RESOLVE, with whom I worked for a number of years and who greatly influenced and shaped my thinking on infertility are Carol Frost Vercollone, M.S.W., and Merle Bombardieri, M.S.W.

The text of this book might have been arid and devoid of feelings were it not for the generous amount of anecdotal material used throughout. For these contributions I cannot name the names I know so well, but I hope each person recognizes his or her value in sharing feelings and experiences that bring heart and soul to this book. These quotes make infertility real to the reader. They bring it home, sometimes with painful impact, in words I never could have found.

Contents

PART II *Psychosocial Aspects of Infertility*

Foreword

In May of 1977, an extraordinary event took place in the field of infertility. A book was published that contained not only the medical and surgical aspects of the problem but also an entire section devoted to its psychosocial impact and the feelings that infertile couples endure. Even more extraordinary was that the author was not a physician specializing in this field, but an infertile woman. That she was also a nurse specialist in maternal–child health provided an excellent background, which lent medical credibility and perspective. But it was her personal experience, first as an infertile woman, and then as a counselor of infertile couples, that added the *human* element to this book. It was a first of its kind, and has stood the test of time as a classic in its field. I believe it to be the best book ever written on the emotional aspects of infertility. When Barbara Eck Menning approached me to be the medical reader for her revision, I was honored. Even with a very busy medical and teaching schedule, I had to find time to help on such a worthy project.

Revision in the field of infertility writing could happen annually, so rapidly does the research, investigation, attempted treatment, and social-ethical-legal picture change. The conservative practitioner trembles as he or she watches the latest "breakthroughs" in extracorporeal conception, gamete transfer, the use of embryo donors, embryo freezing, and surrogate motherhood. While we ache for the plight of the childless couples of this country and this world, one wonders if "a baby at any cost" should be the current trend, and where the ethical and legal guidelines for such decisions are to come from. On the other hand, the past decade has provided many excellent medical and surgical treatments for the infertility specialist's armament, aided by state-of-the-art diagnostic tools to first ascertain the problem. Surely there is more reason for celebration than there is cause for alarm with current advances in the field.

Consumer advocacy organizations such as RESOLVE have assumed a vital role in the education of infertile couples and in cautioning them against voluntary or involuntary exploitation by "quick fixes," fads, gimmickery, and unethical or illegal procedures. Barbara Eck Menning set the tone for the organization when she founded it in 1973. She believed there was no greater need than that of providing the infertile couple with information and emotional support. The organization set out to remain apolitical, nondenominational, and unbiased in its view of what was *right* among the avenues available to couples seeking to achieve pregnancy or to have a family by alternative means. If it was legal—or perhaps we should say, not illegal—then a couple had a right to learn about it. What decision they made they would have to live with. RESOLVE does not make decisions for anyone. This consumer advocacy stance has won RESOLVE the respect of most specialists in this field. I suspect that those who do not subscribe to RESOLVE's excellent newsletter or refer to its support groups are mistakenly threatened by the idea that a consumer organization is somehow preempting their services. In truth, they provide a service that physicians cannot.

It is a wise infertility specialist who realizes that one can give only so much education and emotional support in the course of daily care. We would like to give more, and we are often frustrated because we cannot. Those of us who have referred patients to RESOLVE support groups have benefited from their educated approach to their case, their desire to be full participants, and their demands to be respectfully and carefully managed. RESOLVE support groups allow patients with a variety of problems and from a variety of physicians to exchange information and feelings. I am aware that in the beginning often there are "war stories" about anger at their physicians' handling of the case, miscommunications, and lack of emotional support. But RESOLVE groups are not formed just to encourage anger and catharsis, but to hold each individual and couple responsible for asking for what they need and for trying to achieve it. They are also held accountable for destructive communications and behaviors, which may compound their infertility situation. These couples become better patients by educating themselves and being encouraged to suggest helpful changes in their care. The days of "doctor as God" are over. Doctor as "partner in care" has come of age. We ought to be very grateful.

From the beginning, RESOLVE tried to make change "within the system." I credit Barbara Eck Menning with the wisdom and the patience to work *with* physicians instead of against them in advocating better and more humane care for infertile couples. In the second year of her work with RESOLVE, Barbara received a letter and then a phone call from the American Fertility Society ethics committee, investigating who she was and what services she was offering to infertile couples. Apparently she satisfied them with both her answers and her example, for some years later she was invited to contribute an article to their journal, *Fertility and Sterility* in 1982, and was asked to present a major paper on "Emotional Needs of Infertile Couples" at their 1983 annual convention. To my knowledge, these were firsts on two levels: She was the first nurse ever so honored; and more important, it was the first time emotional aspects of infertility had ever been addressed nonclinically in either forum. She has since completed the program at the Harvard University School of Public Health and has received her M.P.H.

I have been honored to serve RESOLVE for ten years in a variety of capacities, and to know Barbara Eck Menning as a friend and colleague even longer. This new revision of her book presents the reader with the most up-to-date summary of infertility investigation, causes, and treatment. It discusses with unbiased candor the "new technologies." But most of all, it contains an enlarged and expanded section of the psychosocial aspects of infertility and the alternatives available for those who cannot achieve a pregnancy. Also included are helpful coping techniques for stress and marital and sexual conflicts, which are bound to arise. Her bibliography of suggested readings provides ample opportunity for the reader to pursue many aspects of the subject in more depth. I am as enthusiastic about this new book as I was about the original, and I know it will take its place once more as the classic in the field.

—Isaac Schiff, M.D.
Director, Fertility, Endocrine,
and Menopause Unit
Brigham and Women's Hospital
Boston, Massachusetts

Preface

Infertility hurts. I know . . . I am an infertile woman. There was a time, some years ago, when I was not able to say those words at all, much less think of myself as an infertile woman. The words seemed mutually exclusive. I could be either infertile or a woman, but not both. The time of my infertility investigation and attempted treatment was filled with turmoil, both physical and emotional. I did not understand what was happening to me, in spite of a graduate degree in maternal–child health nursing. I did not understand my feelings in spite of the fact that I had counseled others extensively. I did not understand why my family and friends could not share my pain when we were able to communicate about everything else. Most of all, I could not understand why infertility *hurt* so much. After all, I had a career to pursue if I couldn't have children. I was born of a generation doing such liberal things as choosing to cohabit instead of marry, delaying childbearing until the years after thirty-five, and even choosing not to have children at all. The key word here is *choice.* I had *chosen* to marry; I had *chosen* a traditional life-style; I had *chosen* to have children. Infertility robbed me of my right to choose to have my own genetic children.

People who are infertile need help! They can be helped in two distinct ways. They need information, and they need support. The first half of this book is geared to providing information. It addresses the questions of what infertility is, what the common female and male causes of it and treatments for it are, and how to go about finding the best possible medical care in hopes of being among the 50 percent of infertile couples who go on to achieve a successful pregnancy. Acquiring information provides a sense of coping with the loss of control over their lives and destinies that infertile couples experience. There has been a vacuum in writing about infertility until recently. When this manuscript was first published in 1977, there was little between medical articles featuring white-rat research and molecular language and the opposite extreme of sensational and poorly researched stories in popular magazines.

But lack of information has been only half the problem. Lack of understanding, and therefore support, for the infertile couple has been an even greater vacuum. The second half of this book deals with the psychosocial aspects of infertility—or to put it more simply, the *feelings* and their origins and impact. Infertile people and the people who deal with them need to understand why fertility (hence infertility) is such a powerful force in present-day society and why there is still so much pressure upon a married couple to bear children. *Infertility represents not merely an inconvenience, but a major life crisis.* It is filled with painful feelings and shakes to our core our most basic concepts of sexuality, self-image, and self-esteem. The couple who cannot ever successfully conceive or carry a pregnancy to live birth (and half the infertile population will fall in this category) need to understand how to deal with their feelings so that they can work toward a healthy resolution and get on with selection of an alternative—be it adoption, donor insemination, or childfree living.

One in every six couples of childbearing age in this country has an infertility problem—more than 10 million people. Ironically, one of the most common feelings of infertile couples is the isolation of "being all alone." I felt the same way when I was going through my experience. In desperation I turned to individual therapy and found it helpful and reassuring. But how I would have loved to have shared my feelings and have had them validated by others who were infertile! In 1973, because of these feelings, I founded an organization in Boston to offer counseling and support groups to those who were infertile. The organization literally started at my kitchen table but soon became a viable and growing operation. We called the organization RESOLVE because our goal was to help people resolve the infertility situation and the painful feelings surrounding it. Since 1973 RESOLVE, Inc., has grown to be a national organization with more than 40 chapters and thousands of members. During the years from 1973 to 1982, when I served as RESOLVE's executive director, I led 16 support groups, counseled hundreds of individuals and couples, conducted endless hours of phone counseling, edited the newsletter, and collected an enormous file of personal letters, case histories, group notes, and testimonials. This experience has provided the basis for my writing about the psychosocial aspects of infertility. To keep current in medical aspects, I undertook a daily review of the medical literature, attended many seminars, and, toward the end, was conducting training and seminars on this subject.

In 1982, after graduating from Harvard School of Public Health, I left

RESOLVE to pursue other areas of interest. I have remained in very close contact with both the staff and the activities of RESOLVE in these past six years. Infertility will always be a significant issue to me, wherever my life and career may take me. My three adopted multiracial children, who were preschoolers when this book's first edition was published, are now teenagers. Ten years has brought many changes—exciting and somewhat unsettling—to the subject of infertility. It became necessary to revise the medical section of the book completely. A whole new chapter called "New Technologies" had to be added. Ethical, legal, and moral concerns that didn't exist ten years ago are now very much with us. This new and expanded second edition of the original book was mandated by the multitude of changes in therapies and options that the last decade has brought to us. It is the best and most exciting reason to revise a book—because so much has changed!

—Barbara Eck Menning
Cape Cod, Massachusetts

PART I

Medical Aspects
of Infertility

1. What Is Infertility?

Multiplication is vexation,
Division is as bad.
The Rule of Three doth puzzle me,
And Practice drives me mad.

MOTHER GOOSE RHYME

People have never been more in control of their lives. Environment, food, shelter, disease, reproduction—most natural forces seem to bend to human will. For better or worse we attempt to control things.

The control of reproduction has been a major social trend in America since World War II. The condom and foam of the prewar generation gave way to the diaphragm of the postwar 1940s, only to be replaced by the Pill and the IUD of the 1960s and 1970s. Couples can now have active and spontaneous sexual relations, secure in the knowledge that their birth control measure is almost 100 percent effective. For the occasional error, therapeutic abortion remains as a backup measure. Many American families now plan their families as meticulously as they do their major financial investments, a move to a new location, or a career change—measuring all the pros and cons and waiting until all the elements are just exactly right:

Six years ago my husband and I got married; we knew that children would definitely be part of our life. This we did not question. What we did discuss was *when*. We decided to wait a year or two to let me use my college degree, buy a house, and establish a good foundation before we brought children into the world. We wanted everything to be just right for the challenging job of parenting.

Here I sit six years later with my husband, established roots, a house, years of teaching experience . . . and no children.

THE PRESUMPTION OF FERTILITY

Fertility (in the woman) is defined as the ability to conceive and give birth to a live baby or (in the man) the ability to impregnate a woman. By its very definition, fertility can be known only after the fact. Until a pregnancy occurs, a man and woman may believe they are fertile, based on family precedents or the odds in general. But they cannot *know* they are fertile until a conception and live birth have occurred. This is equally true of those who have had previous births or abortions. Past fertility tells nothing about present fertility. Fertility is not a life force that may be turned on at will. Although it is true that pregnancy may be prevented with almost 100 percent certainty, it is also true that once birth control measures are stopped, 15 percent of all couples will experience some degree of infertility.

DEFINITION OF INFERTILITY

Infertility is defined as *the inability to conceive a pregnancy after a year or more of regular sexual relations without contraception, or the inability to carry pregnancies to a live birth*. It is estimated that 15 percent of the population of childbearing age in America is infertile at any given time. *This amounts to 1 in every 6 couples of childbearing age—more than 10 million people in this country alone.*

Infertility is further classified as either *primary*, when there is no previous history of pregnancy, or *secondary*, when it occurs after one or more successful pregnancies. The medical term *sterility* is often misused. Technically, it should be reserved for cases of permanent and incurable infertility. The euphemism *subfertility* has been seen in the literature lately, connoting those individuals or couples who have a borderline problem. To eliminate confusion, the term *infertility* will be used throughout this book, as it most correctly encompasses all states of the inability to conceive or carry pregnancy.

COMMON MYTHS ABOUT INFERTILITY

In order to define infertility, it is first necessary to debunk some old myths and say what it is *not:*

1. *Infertility is not a "female condition."* It surprises most people to learn that in almost half of all cases of infertility, a male problem is found. A breakdown of infertility by cause reveals a female problem in 35 percent of cases, a male problem in 35 percent, a combined problem of the couple in 20 percent, and unknown problems in the remaining 10 percent.

2. *Infertility is not usually due to psychological factors.* A physical problem is found in 90 percent of all infertility cases that have been thoroughly investigated by a qualified doctor. The stress and emotions an infertile couple may exhibit are the *result* of their infertility, not the *cause* of it.

3. *Infertility is not always incurable.* Between 40 and 50 percent of those couples who enter a proper investigation of their problem will respond to treatment with a successful pregnancy. Some types of problems respond with higher success rates; some are much lower. Those who do not seek help have a "spontaneous cure rate" of about 10 percent after a year of infertility and 5 percent after two years.

4. *Infertility is not a sexual disorder.* Infertility has nothing to do with the ability to perform normally in sexual relations in the vast majority of cases. Infertile men and women are capable of experiencing the same spectrum of physical and emotional sexual responses as are other couples.

5. *If you adopt a baby, you'll get pregnant.* This is one of the most painful myths for infertile couples to deal with. First, it suggests that adoption is only a means to an end, not an end in itself. Second, it is simply not true! Dr. Emmett Lamb studied a large sample of infertile couples who came through the clinic at Stanford University. He compared pregnancy rates of couples who chose to adopt with those who did not. The study revealed a "spontaneous cure rate" of 5 percent in either case.

6. *Infertility is nature's way of controlling population.* Zero population growth is an admirable cause in a time of world overpopulation, but it still allows a couple to replace themselves with two children. Those who wish to be childfree by choice or to raise single children have the right to do so. Infertility, for those who desire children, is a denial of the right to choose.

INFERTILITY ON THE INCREASE

There is growing concern that certain sociological, environmental, and medical factors are resulting in increasing numbers of infertile couples. Young men and women are sexually active at younger ages and often have multiple partners. This greatly increases the risk of sexually transmitted diseases (venereal disease). The recent appearance of new drug-resistant strains of gonorrhea and of chlamydia and ureaplasma infections has complicated diagnosis and treatment. The AIDS epidemic is of great concern for the mortality rate; and its concern in connection with fertility is in the use of donor semen for achieving pregnancy. A major factor in the infertility increase has been delaying marriage and attempting childbearing in the years after thirty and even thirty-five. The longer men and women live, the greater their chance for developing disease. Not only are women less fertile after the age of thirty, but they may have reduced fertility as a result of their having used birth control. Some clinics report seeing increasing numbers of women who do not ovulate spontaneously after going off the birth control pill. The IUD has been associated with as much as a 10 percent risk of infection. Even therapeutic abortion may be associated with 1 to 5 percent risk of infection and may cause trauma to the cervix in very young women, or to the cells that produce cervical mucus. Women over thirty are much more likely to have symptoms of endometriosis—a major infertility problem.

"Life-style" changes in the past decade have included more use of so-called recreational drugs such as marijuana and cocaine as well as continued use of alcohol and cigarettes. Environmentally we are concerned about exposure to chemicals in our food, our drinking water, and the very air we breathe. Even women's breast milk has been found unsafe for consumption in some communities. Males are much more at risk for infertility because of drugs and pollutants, since they are constantly forming sperm cells, while women are born with their entire egg supply. Alarming studies have shown a decrease in sperm counts over the past 30 years to almost half of what was found to be "normal" then.

PREVENTION OF INFERTILITY

The average American adolescent still gets relatively little preparation for coping with his or her developing sexuality. In some school systems, and in some homes and churches, careful and thoughtful time is given to the issues of bodily and emotional changes, the facts of reproduction and contraception, and responsible behavior for the sexually active person. Infertility is rarely mentioned as a consequence of willful or negligent misuse of one's body or lack of information about factors that might put certain people at risk. Some very important information ought to be shared in any comprehensive sexual education program about measures that may help ensure future fertility:

1. Any person who is sexually active, especially with multiple partners, should be alert to the signs of infection in the reproductive tract.

Symptoms may include discharge from the vagina or urethra, pain during urination, low-grade fever, chancre (open sores) of the genitals, pelvic tenderness or pain in women, and rashes. The woman is much more likely to contract sexually transmitted disease that can effect future fertility. Because the first portion of a man's reproductive system is involved with his urinary tract, frequent flushing of the urethra makes ascending infection far less likely. Also, the man is more likely to have early bothersome symptoms, whereas the woman frequently is asymptomatic until significant reproductive damage is done. If one partner is found to have an infection, *both* must be treated.

2. The choice of a birth control method should be made very carefully. The IUD, with its associated infection rate, is no longer on the market in the United States—primarily because of litigation against manufacturers for its harmful side effects—except for the Progestasert. It is best reserved for women who have completed their childbearing. The Pill should be prescribed cautiously for very young women who have erratic menstrual patterns. Women who recover menstrual function quickly after stopping the Pill are those who had normal cycles before they began the Pill. It is also suggested now that the duration of time a woman remains on the Pill is not likely to affect future fertility, but that women who go on and off the Pill have more problems regaining normal ovulation. Barrier methods used along with spermicidal jelly such as the condom or the diaphragm or cervical cap are free of risks to future fertility but are often less desirable to sexually active young people because they are not as conducive to spontaneous sex. They also carry a slight risk of unplanned pregnancy. Abstinence should be included in any discussion of birth control as the method with the least risks and 100 percent protection.

3. The decision to have a therapeutic abortion should be made very carefully if unplanned pregnancy does arise. Careful cervical dilation in a young woman is important to her future fertility. Any postabortion symptoms of infection—foul discharge, pelvic tenderness, fever— should be reported immediately to the doctor. Women who undergo repeated abortions as a result of not using birth control, or using it incorrectly, are at more risk for future infertility problems. This is irresponsible behavior for a sexually active person, but if the community and/or family have denied a woman access to sexual education they are equally at fault.

4. All young boys should now be immunized against mumps long before puberty to protect against mumps orchitis (inflammation of a testis) which can lead to infertility. Young men involved in sports should wear proper protective gear such as athletic supporters or cups to

prevent injury to the scrotum or torsion of the testicles. Undescended testicles in the male are now surgically descended well before puberty. Undescended testicles are still an important risk factor for future fertility as well as for cancer of the testicle. History of childhood hernia surgery is also significant, because of the proximity of important blood vessels to the testes. Finally, diethylstilbestrol (DES) exposure in utero is a risk factor for men as well as women.

5. Young women who menstruate very erratically or cease to menstruate for long spells, or those who have a family history of endometriosis, may be at risk for future fertility problems. A history of a ruptured appendix is frequently associated with scarring and adhesions in the pelvic cavity, which may impair fertility. DES exposure in utero may result in structural problems of the uterus and tubes and it also needs close monitoring for an increased risk of vaginal cancer.

6. Women who choose to delay childbearing into the years after age thirty, and especially after thirty-five are up against a biological time clock. If a problem with fertility is found that can be treated, they simply have less time to wait patiently for a pregnancy. A woman is also at increased risk after thirty-five for certain genetic defects of her baby (Down's syndrome being the most common). Many doctors will recommend amniocentesis for all patients over thirty-five. Finally, if a problem with fertility is found but cannot be successfully treated, the couple involved may have missed the chance to adopt an infant. Many agencies will not place an infant in a home with parents over forty years, and the wait for some types of adoption may be three to five years.

2. The Human Reproductive System

*The universe resounds with the joyful
cry, I am!*

To understand infertility, and the tests and treatments associated with it, the reader should first be familiar with the normal reproductive anatomy and physiology of both the man and the woman. Words or phrases that are unfamiliar and not defined in the text can be looked up in the glossary at the end of the book.

THE MALE REPRODUCTIVE SYSTEM

The male reproductive system consists of the testes and a system of excretory ducts and their accessory structures (see fig. 1). In descending order these organs include the *testes,* a pair of oval bodies lying in the scrotal sac. This location outside the body cavity keeps the testes slightly cooler than body temperature (about 2°), which is vital to sperm production. This temperature is maintained carefully by the scrotal muscles, which contract to bring the testes closer to the body in cold weather and relax to drop the testes away from the body in warm weather. The testes have two major functions: to produce the male sex hormone, testosterone, and to produce sperm cells. The male does not function in a cycle as the female does. From puberty on, his production of sperm and hormones remains relatively constant, whether or

FRONTAL VIEW

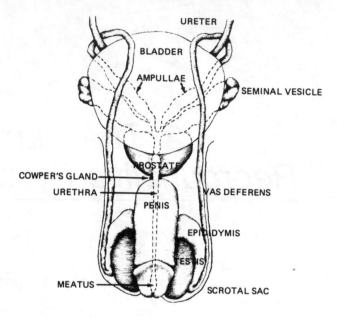

CROSS-SECTION

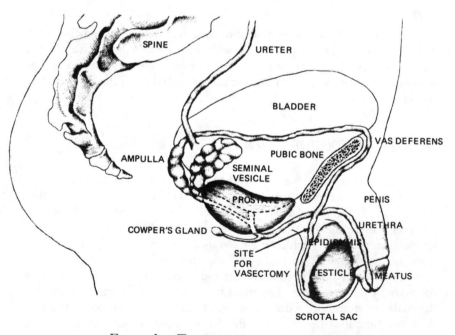

FIGURE 1. THE MALE REPRODUCTIVE SYSTEM

not he is sexually active. It takes approximately 74 days for the testes to produce sperm cells. Then the still immature sperm are passed slowly through a long coiled tube called the *epididymis*, where they undergo maturation and achieve motility (the ability to move) for about one more week. Connected to the epididymis are two long ducts called the *vasa deferentia* (singular, *vas deferens*). The bottom end of the vas deferens, where it leaves the epididymis, is the site of a vasectomy in males who undergo sterilization. The thick-walled vas deferens is in a constant state of muscular action that gently "squeezes" sperm along the way to where the tube widens out to form the *ampullae*. Some sperm are stored here prior to ejaculation, although the majority are stored in the epididymis. Just beyond the ampullae are two offshoots of the vasa deferentia, called the *seminal vesicles*. These glands are important for their production of the sugar fructose, which is needed as fuel by the sperm for their long journey.

Just beyond the seminal vesicles, at the base of the bladder, lies the *prostate gland*, which contributes most of the actual seminal fluid and an important chemical or enzyme that causes the semen to liquify from its coagulated state shortly after ejaculation. The secretion of the prostate is highly alkaline to neutralize the acidity of the urethra and the woman's vagina. Beyond the prostate, situated at the base of the penile shaft in the urethra, are a pair of small glands, called *Cowper's glands*, which add a small amount of lubricant to the seminal fluid before ejaculation takes place. Finally, there is the *penis*, the organ of copulation, by means of which the man deposits the seminal fluid into the vagina of the woman. The penis contains cavernous spaces that have the capacity to fill with blood when stimulated, which results in erection and rigidity of the organ for intercourse.

The following sequence will further illustrate the event that takes place during intercourse. Sperm are produced in the testes, matured in the epididymis, and stored in the ampullae. At the time of excitation, the vasa deferentia increase their upward contractions, sending more sperm into the ampullae. Upon ejaculation, the seminal vesicles, the prostate, and the Cowper's gland all add their secretions to the sperm, making semen or seminal fluid. The ejaculate is discharged into the vagina through the erect penis. A normal ejaculate contains anywhere from 40 to 150 million highly active sperm in about 2 to 5 cc of semen. Only about 2 percent of the ejaculate is actually sperm cells. Once deposited in the vagina, only about 10 percent of the sperm will actually survive to penetrate the cervical mucus and begin the long swim toward an ovum.

THE FEMALE REPRODUCTIVE SYSTEM

The reproductive system of the female is entirely internal, in contrast to that of the male (see fig. 2). The organs and glands, in ascending order, are the

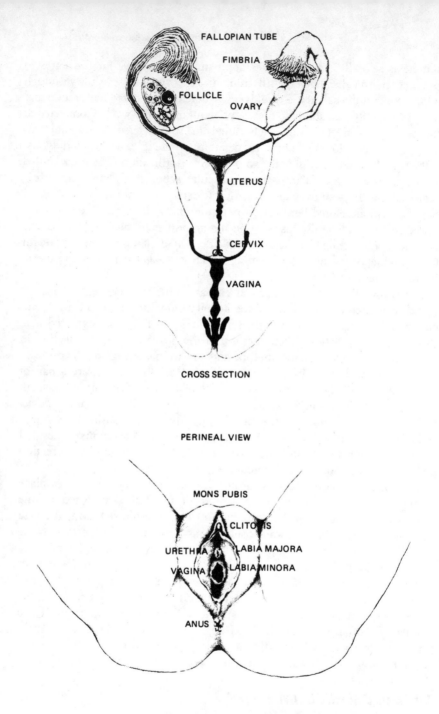

FIGURE 2.   THE FEMALE REPRODUCTIVE SYSTEM

vagina, a passage lined with mucous membrane about 3 to 5 inches in length and capable of great expansion. The vagina opens into the vulva, which is not a particular organ but a series of folds that protect the vagina. These external genital structures include the *mons pubis*, the outer and inner lips (*labia majora* and *minora*), the *clitoris*, the *hymen* (if intact), the *urethra*, and two pairs of lubricating glands. The vagina leads upward to a blind vault into which the *cervix* projects. The cervix is a fibrous plug of tissue, sometimes called the "neck of the uterus." It has a narrow opening (*cervical os*), and its mucous lining and crypts produce abundant secretions that can vary from an impassable mucus plug to watery elastic strands, depending on the time in a woman's cycle and the hormones being produced. The mucus plug is vital to protecting the woman from ascending infections, to which she is much more vulnerable than is the man.

Above the cervix lies the *uterus*, a thick-walled muscular organ about the size and shape of a pear in the nonpregnant state, but capable of expanding more than 40 times this size in pregnancy. The cavity of the uterus is triangular in shape, widest at the top (fundus) and narrow at the cervical end. The nonpregnant uterus can contain only a teaspoon of liquid comfortably. The uterus is lined with mucous membrane called *endometrium*, which waxes and wanes under the influence of the hormones a woman secretes.

The *fallopian tubes* are two trumpet-shaped, flexible, muscular tubes about 4 inches long that arise off the fundus, one to each side. At the inner portion, the tubes have a diameter narrower than a lead pencil. The tubes reach upward and slightly behind the uterus. They are lined with membrane containing tiny hairlike projections (*cilia*) which move with the contraction of the musculature of the tubes to produce a progressive wave to "sweep" the ovum toward the uterus. In addition, the tubes contain secretions that affect sperm-egg interaction. The outermost end of the fallopian tubes are called the *fimbriated ends*. These are flared and contain fringed projections thought to "catch" the ovum after ovulation and draw it into the tube. The ovary is not directly connected to the tube. Below the fimbriated ends lie the *ovaries*, one on each side. Ovaries are about the size of walnuts and have two important functions: to produce the female hormones estrogen and progesterone, and to produce a ripened ovum once each menstrual cycle. The ovaries do not alternate consistently and the monthly egg may come from either side. In cases where a woman has only one ovary, it takes over monthly ovulation as well as the entire production of hormones.

THE MENSTRUAL CYCLE

A woman's body operates in a cyclical manner from the onset of her menstruation (menarche) to its cessation (menopause). Although women's cycles vary greatly in length, the sequence of events in an idealized 28-day cycle (see fig. 3) follows this course: The first day of the cycle is the first day of *menstruation*, the shedding of the lining of the uterus from the previous cycle. Throughout the cycle, the pituitary, a small gland at the base of the brain, dependent upon the hypothalamus, sends out *follicular stimulating hormone* (FSH), which stimulates the ovary to ripen a follicle and mature an ovum. Another hormone, *luteinizing hormone* (LH), is produced by the pituitary in somewhat higher amounts throughout the cycle. A large surge of LH that occurs right before ovulation is thought to help release the mature ovum at ovulation time. Close monitoring of blood and urine levels for this surge has helped enormously in pinpointing ovulation. Throughout the entire cycle, the ovary is producing estrogen. The "peak" of estrogen produced just prior to ovulation is responsible for turning cervical mucus from an impassable plug to watery elastic strands which sperm can penetrate easily.

Ovulation takes place on about the fourteenth day from the first day of menstruation. The tiny ovum is extruded from the ovary and, with luck, is picked up by the fringed projections of the fimbriated end of the fallopian tube nearest the ovary and swept along into the tube. If fertilization is to take place, it occurs in the outer third of the tube, within 12 to 24 hours after ovulation. Meanwhile, the ruptured follicle that produced the ovum now becomes a functioning gland called the *corpus luteum*, named for its yellow luteal lining. The gland now produces the hormone *progesterone*, in addition to *estrogen*, which prepares the uterus with a lush secretory lining needed for implantation in case fertilization has occurred.

If the ovum has been fertilized, the tiny mass of slowly dividing cells floats freely down the fallopian tube and into the uterus, where it implants in the lining about 6 days after ovulation (day 20 of the cycle). Once implanted in the uterus, the conceptus develops a feedback mechanism with the corpus luteum, telling it to go on producing progesterone, thus preventing menstruation and preserving the lining and the pregnancy. This message is sent by the cells that are destined to become the placenta, and the "messenger" is the hormone that pregnancy tests measure, *human chorionic gonadotropin* (HCG). The placenta is not capable of taking over progesterone production from the corpus luteum for almost two months.

If fertilization has not occurred, the ovum passes into the uterus and the corpus luteum fails to receive the signal to continue progesterone production. In this case, on about the twenty-sixth day of the cycle, the corpus luteum deteriorates into a nonfunctioning gland and the progesterone level falls. The uterus begins to break down its rich lining and sloughs it off. The next menstrual period begins within several days.

It is important to point out that women may have menstruation even though they have not ovulated. It is thought that many women have such

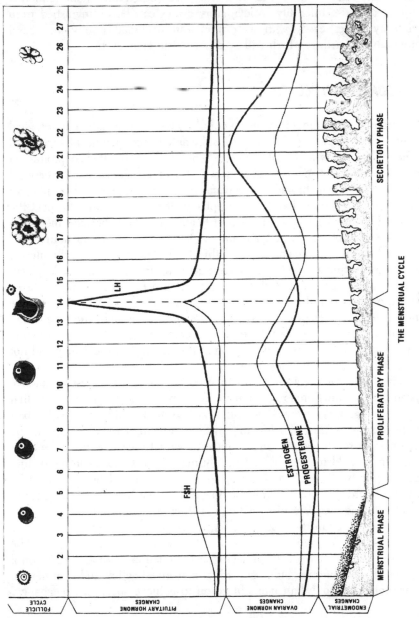

FIGURE 3. AN IDEALIZED 28-DAY MENSTRUAL CYCLE

anovulatory cycles from time to time, and some women have them frequently enough to cause infertility. Anovulatory cycles can be distinguished from ovulatory cycles easily with a combination of blood testing and basal temperature charting, which will be discussed in chapter 4.

HOW CONCEPTION OCCURS

The premise of fertility in any given couple is based on specific physiological events and their timing. The man must be able to produce healthy sperm of sufficient numbers and motility. The woman must be able to produce a healthy ovum. The sperm must be deposited in the vagina, near the cervical opening, and swim through the cervical mucus to the end of the fallopian tube. The ovum must have been swept into the tube in order to meet the sperm. Timing of sexual relations is critically important, because the ovum may live as briefly as 12 to 24 hours, and the sperm 24 to 48 hours. The fertilized ovum must be able to move through the tube and enter the uterus, where it must find a lining of sufficient quality for implantation to take place. The feedback mechanism with the corpus luteum must begin and continue for almost two months, until the developing placenta of the fetus is large enough to take over progesterone production and maintain the pregnancy. The uterus must be structurally sound and capable of great expansion, while the cervix must be strong enough to hold the developing pregnancy and not dilate until the fetus is ready to be born.

Considering the precision with which both male and female reproductive systems must function to result in a live birth, it seems miraculous that human beings are conceived and born at all! Human fertility is assured in part by the reliable excesses of nature in providing more than 400 ovulations in the lifetime of a fertile woman and abundant sperm to fertilize any ovum in a fertile man. Add to this the fact that humans, unlike lower forms of life, demonstrate willingness and desire to have sexual relations frequently, without regard to the season or to the time of a woman's cycle. Consequently, couples having sexual relations without birth control can expect a 25 percent rate of pregnancy in the first cycle, 60 percent of such couples would have conceived by six months, and 85 percent by the end of one year. The remaining 15 percent of couples having sexual relations without birth control may be termed infertile, although with proper investigation and treatment of their problem, more than half will go on to achieve successful pregnancy.

3. Selecting Your Doctor

It's easy finding reasons why other folks should be patient.

GEORGE ELIOT

ADAM BEDE

WHEN IS A COUPLE INFERTILE?

Because infertility is a *dynamic* state of being unable to conceive or carry a pregnancy, there is a practical problem of deciding just when a couple should consider themselves infertile. Although infertility has been defined as inability to conceive or carry pregnancy after a year of effort, it often unfolds to a couple in gradual fashion, progressing from small doubts to deeper concern and intensification of the search for answers and a "cure." The labyrinth of infertility may take years to negotiate, or it may only be a matter of a few simple tests and treatment. One never knows until the process is begun.

Couples often resist the label "infertile" or feel ambivalent applying the term to themselves. Frequently a couple cannot embark on a search for the problem until they are able to accept that they might, indeed, be infertile. For one couple this might be after only three or four months without achieving a pregnancy; for another couple it could take three or four years. Some individuals remain childless forever and still resist calling themselves infertile. This underscores the strength of society's negative attitude toward infertility, even in a time when birth control, abortion, and vasectomies are freely discussed.

17

After our first appointment I remember telling myself I should be relieved that the doctor had taken our problem seriously and was going to do something about it. But when I got home and tried to tell my husband what had happened, I started crying and couldn't get a word out. Finally I realized that the problem was that by beginning tests, we were now admitting we had an infertility problem and I didn't want to. I wanted pregnancy to be natural and spontaneous, and now I knew it wouldn't be.

Statistics have shown that about 85 percent of couples who are not using birth control will conceive within one year of effort. This makes a convincing argument for a couple to attempt a pregnancy for at least a year before considering themselves infertile. Many doctors will not proceed with an infertility investigation until a year goes by, and some feel two years is a necessary trial before tests are begun. The trouble with statistics and "necessary trials" is that they are not geared to the individual needs of people. Some couples want to begin working actively on the problem almost from the first month, just as some feel the need to postpone, ignore, or deny the problem for extended periods of time. It seems reasonable that the couple, not the doctor, should decide when they are anxious enough to begin an investigation. The doctor can advise the couple of the chances for spontaneous pregnancy in the first year but should not make light of their feelings or send them away with platitudes.

We had been trying for maybe seven months and I was already a basket case— convinced we would never have children, weepy at every period. I made an appointment with a gynecologist who is supposed to be good at these things. The whole visit was a nightmare. He totally refused to listen to me and kept assuring me that I was "normal as blueberry pie" and would be "nicely pregnant" in no time. After the pelvic, he sat me down in his office, peered over his glasses at me, and prescribed—yes, I mean he literally ordered—that I take a warm shower and glass of sherry every night before bedtime and make love "as often as possible!"

Even if a couple becomes anxious after only six months of effort, there is no harm in allowing them to come in for examinations (a pelvic for the woman, a urologic exam for the man). The woman can be instructed to start charting her basal temperature (see pages 28 to 31). The man can have a semen analysis (see pages 39 to 41). If the initial tests are normal, the woman can chart her cycle for five or six months and the couple will have completed their year of effort with the preliminary phase of investigation well under way with little expense and no incurred tests that carry risk. It is true that the spontaneous cure rate in early infertility cases is high. Doctors will often lose these couples as patients within a few months to the happy announcement of pregnancy. However, it is also true that a simple problem may be found and corrected during this time that will save a couple months of time and anxiety in their quest to become parents.

Some couples are justified in having an early concern about infertility. The most obvious category is anyone over thirty-five years old, since there is a definite social trend in America toward delaying marriage and childbearing into the years after thirty. While it is economically, sociologically, and psychologically sound for couples to follow and be part of this trend, a woman's reproductive system is maximally fertile when she is in her mid-twenties, and her fertility gradually tapers off to when she is thirty and declines more rapidly after that. Studies have shown that the time required to conceive a wanted child increases with age and the risk of being unable to bear a child seems to rise from about 5 percent at ages twenty to twenty-four to as much as 16 percent when a woman is thirty to thirty-five.*

Men or women who have identified risk factors to fertility (see chapter 1) are also among those who should not wait for a "year of effort" before seeing a doctor. They are justified in seeking help early and may even go so far as having premarital examinations, especially if childbearing is a very important motive for the marriage.

CHOOSING A DOCTOR

When the time finally comes that a couple decide "something is wrong," where should they turn for help? Because infertility is most often thought of as a "woman's problem," most couples begin by seeing a gynecologist or family physician. While this may be an adequate starting place, too often there is a tendency to be loyal to the first doctor seen, allowing an entire investigation to progress (in some fashion) even though the doctor does not have specialized skills in infertility. Doctors would do their patients a great service if they observed logical points of referral to their colleagues who are specialists. In chapter 4 these referral points will be discussed in greater depth.

An *infertility specialist* is a doctor who has added to his or her basic residency in obstetrics and gynecology a subspecialty fellowship in reproductive endocrinology and infertility. Endocrinology/infertility was not recognized as a subspecialty subject for board certification until 1974. In the five years from 1974 through 1978, a total of 64 physicians received this board certification. In 1987 this number had increased to 231.† This three-year

---

* Jane Menken, James Trussell, and Ulla Larsen, "Age and Infertility," *Science*, September 26, 1986, p. 1393.

† Reported by the American Board of Obstetrics and Gynecologists.

additional training qualifies the doctor to manage all but surgical investigation and treatment of the male, which is referred to a urologist. There are still relatively few infertility specialists and they are generally concentrated in major medical centers in large cities. Some devote most of their time to research and don't see patients. A list of the specialists in your area can be obtained from RESOLVE. The American Fertility Society, a membership organization of doctors, will also provide lists of specialists, but it will not make specific recommendations. One important feature of a specialist is that he or she will usually not carry an obstetrical caseload or will limit it to severely high-risk patients. This is important and necessary, since the doctor who combines obstetrics and infertility is invariably at the mercy of the obstetrical patients, often at the expense of the infertile couples.

> I was having husband insemination and had strict orders to come to the office with a very fresh semen specimen—within 30 minutes if possible. When I arrived, the receptionist said that the doctor was out delivering a baby. I waited a long time and I finally asked if one of the other doctors could do the insemination. The nurse said no, since our doctor could not be reached by phone. In the meantime the specimen began to leak through the bag. I was in a waiting room packed with pregnant women and tried not to cry, but I was not successful. The whole episode was awful!

Most infertility specialists prefer to see the couple together on the first visit. Many couples use this first visit simply to "interview" the specialist and to see if the policies and milieu of the practice are going to meet their emotional, financial, and physical needs. The ideal infertility practice utilizes a team approach with a reproductive endocrinologist, a urologist (a new subspecialty dealing just with male infertility is known as *andrology*), a genetic counselor, an infertility counselor, and complete support services for laboratory testing. It is important to emphasize that the infertile couple just starting out may not need all these facilities, but that they should know these exist and that they are indicated for proper management of anything beyond the most routine testing and treatment.

Here are some guidelines that RESOLVE recommends to help the infertile couple locate the proper infertility specialist closest to their location:

1. Call or write RESOLVE (see page 189) to locate the names of specialists located nearest to you. If you are in a very rural area, it may be necessary to travel some distance. In the long run, this may still be less expensive and time-consuming than using a less expert local physician.
2. Plan to attend your first session as a couple. Bring a list of questions

such as: Does the doctor maintain an obstetrical practice? (The answer should be no or very limited.) What is the doctor's additional training that qualifies him or her to be called a "specialist"? Please note that membership in an organization such as the American Fertility Society, while it indicates interest in this area, is simply a membership open to all doctors.

3. Ask how the male and female aspects of infertility are generally managed. Ideally there should be management of both in the same facility, with a very close communication among the various doctors.

4. Find out what supportive counseling services are available to you if you enter this undertaking. Some procedures, such as donor insemination or in vitro fertilization, are extremely taxing and require both screening before they are begun and support throughout the attempt at pregnancy.

5. Finally, most doctors today recognize a well-informed couple as their partners in the rigors of infertility investigation and treatment. The burden is on the couple to be well read and curious about their case, and upon the doctor to welcome the discussion and questions that such a partnership will foster.

YOUR RIGHTS IN THE DOCTOR-PATIENT RELATIONSHIP

The infertile couple should learn to expect some very reasonable rights when they begin to deal with their doctor. By having these, they can reduce the sense of embarrassment and loss of control over their bodies that infertility investigation and treatment may impose.

The normal nonpregnant woman has probably been seeing a gynecologist about once a year for a pelvic exam. The woman entering an infertility investigation will see her doctor several times a month or more, depending on where the problem lies. Examination of her internal reproductive organs requires a woman to assume a graceless position on her back with her legs spread-eagled in stirrups. Even the most gentle and routine procedures are accompanied by a sense of invasion of her private parts that makes any composure and conversation very difficult.

A man may fare little better. While most women are used to examinations of their reproductive organs, most men have never experienced this, unless they have had occasion to have a prostate probed through the rectum. There are relatively few diagnostic procedures for the male and they are largely noninvasive, but they are intensely embarrassing since they deal with close inspection of the sexual organs and microscopic inspection of the seminal fluid. Therefore, it is safe to say both the man and the woman enter the doctor-patient relationship feeling unequal and intimidated by the unknown.

The following list of patient rights needs a brief explanation. A *right* is any situation that would be recognized as legal if the case were brought before a court of law. This list is adapted from several sources, among them a model patients' bill of rights developed by George Annas for the American Civil Liberties Union. This list applies to hospitals and clinics and not to doctors in private practice. If rights are violated in a private practice, the patient has the recourse of seeking another opinion.

Any patient, male or female, should expect the following rights from a concerned doctor:

1. You have the right to be seen fully clothed in the doctor's office to discuss your case and ask questions before you are seen in the examination room. If this is your first visit to the doctor, you may request just an office visit and no examination, to see how you like the doctor and whether you can establish a good relationship.
2. You have the right to be seen on time or to be given an indication of the approximate wait you may have in case of an emergency or unpredictable delay. Clinics can be especially negligent in this area. Your time is important, too!
3. You have the right to be treated respectfully, to be called by your proper name, and to have all interviewing and record taking done in privacy.
4. You have the right to know exactly what each procedure will cost before it is done and whether or not it is covered by insurance. (Since insurance coverage varies widely, you may have to research this yourself.) You have a right to the highest degree of care available without regard to the source of payment.
5. You have a right to be talked to in language you clearly understand. Sometimes the doctor may be guilty of "talking over your head" in your own language. If you speak another language, you have a right to have an interpreter present. This is a service available at most larger medical centers.
6. You have the right to have everything explained to you before the doctor does it. He or she should explain the reason for the procedure, whether it will hurt, any possible side effects, and the results (or when the results will be available).
7. You have the right to know the name and dosage of any medication or solution given to you and the reason for any specimen taken from you, and the results, when known.
8. You have the right to know your temperature, pulse, respiration rate, and blood pressure, and the interpretation of other physical findings made on your case.

9. You have the right to be examined without a drape, if you wish, or to be draped in such a way that you can see what is happening. Some doctors have special mirrors and lights to allow you to see everything they are doing.

10. You have the right to be informed of any research studies to be performed on you and of any students of the health professions being assigned to your case. You may refuse either. If you accept, you have a right to full information about what either will involve.

11. You have the right to make your own decisions about your body. The doctor can only make recommendations. If you are unsure, get a second or even a third opinion.

12. You have the right to have all consent forms and documents fully explained to you before you sign them. You should never sign anything while under medication that could affect your judgment. You should never sign anything under pressure or duress.

13. You have a right to all the information contained in your medical record. You should be able to examine this record upon request.

14. You have the right to change doctors if you feel it is necessary to get the level of care you require. You have the right to a summary of your record and all pertinent X rays or studies being forwarded to your new doctor at your written request. There may be a small charge for the copying and mailing charges to do this. If you are leaving a doctor for a specific reason, you owe it to future patients to inform the doctor of your reason and to suggest ways the doctor might improve his or her practice.

It would be unfair to many fine doctors to imply that patient's rights are violated willfully or maliciously. For example, many doctors withhold information to spare a patient needless worry. They don't tell a patient a test is going to hurt because the patient may tense up. They don't disclose a possible drug side effect for fear of "suggesting" it. Some doctors really believe that women patients are comforted by the paternalistic approach. Others use familiarity or attempts at humor to try to set the patient at ease. The doctor-patient relationship should be the same as any other service-consumer situation. If you feel dissatisfied with either your physical or emotional management, you should discuss it. If the doctor is unwilling or unable to comply with your needs, you have a right to take your business elsewhere.

Communication is so important in the doctor-patient relationship that it deserves special emphasis. It is common for patients to blame themselves for not understanding medical terminology, abbreviations, anatomy and physiology, names of medications, and so forth. While all patients should try to be informed consumers, it is the doctor or nurse who should attempt to explain things to the patient's level of understanding. This is often done by asking the patient to repeat the message back or by asking questions. The patient must be willing to ask for further clarification; the doctor or nurse must be patient enough to give this extra time and attention. Add to this the high level of anxiety that may attend certain procedures and the fact that patients will often hear selectively at such times or have complete or partial memory lapses in such a state. It is imperative that the doctor or nurse repeat important points or even have the patient write them down. The patient who is highly anxious and has issues to discuss with the doctor should always bring in a written list. Communication is a two-way street. *What was said can be valuable only if it was heard, and if it was understood.*

4. Investigation of Infertility

*Be patient toward all that is unsolved
in your heart. . . .
Try to love the questions themselves.*

RILKE

*T*he couple embarking on an infertility workup do so with very mixed emotions. On the one hand there is the relief and excitement of finally acknowledging a problem and taking active control over it. On the other hand there is fear of the unknown physical, emotional, and financial toll this investigation may take. Finally, it may pinpoint a problem in one or the other of the partners and cause fears of "blame" or even abandonment to occur.

It cannot be overstressed that infertility is a problem a *couple* experience together. A single person may have an infertility problem, but it takes a man and woman to conceive a child. In these days of new technologies, perhaps it should more correctly be stated that it takes sperm and an ovum. The vast majority of cases of infertility involve a couple in a committed relationship who long to have a child or children. Therefore they should enter the infertility investigation together, offering support and comfort to each other as they work to fulfill this mutual life goal.

For the sake of convenience, we will separate the female and male aspects of the infertility investigation. The sequence of tests may vary slightly from doctor to doctor, but it usually begins with tests easiest and lowest in risk, and progresses to surgical procedures if necessary. If either the woman or the man has been found "normal" early in the investigation, it still makes good sense to look at the fertility status of that partner periodically, especially if the testing of the other partner is protracted. Fertility fluctuates in both the male and the female and there is no guarantee that one partner is "off the hook" while the other is being investigated. It is precisely this fact that *nothing* can be taken for granted that makes infertility investigation both extremely challenging to the specialist and very frustrating as well.

INVESTIGATION OF THE WOMAN

History and Physical

A thorough and unhurried history taking and general physical can reveal many things to the astute doctor while establishing a basis in communication and caring with the patient. Some history taking may occur with the couple together, but it is imperative that the doctor provide a private setting for each to discuss sensitive issues such as sexual experience and history of previous pregnancies. Some couples have secrets from each other, and it is not unusual for them to differ on issues of sexual satisfaction within the marriage. The doctor usually begins the woman's sexual history with questions about her menstrual history. The age of onset and character of periods may reveal important data. The doctor will ask about any significant illnesses or surgeries. For example, a history of a ruptured appendix in a female is very important to her possible fertility status. Then the doctor will ask about sexual experience before the marriage and the use of any form of birth control. It is vital for the doctor to know if there have been any previous conceptions and whether they resulted in abortion or in birth. The doctor will want to know if the woman has ever experienced a sexually transmitted disease, and if so, what it was and how it was treated. Finally, the doctor should ask some careful psychosexual questions. Was the patient ever the victim of sexual abuse in childhood? Does she have any guilt feelings over sexual encounters in her past or in the present relationship? How would she describe her current sexual activity, in regard to frequency, her ability to lubricate and achieve orgasm, and her feelings toward her partner's sensitivity to her needs? Are they able to communicate openly on such matters? While orgasm is not a prerequisite for fertility in the woman, it may provide insight into the sexual relationship of the couple. Does the couple use any artificial lubricants? (These are likely to be spermicidal.)

Not all doctors have the ability to ask these questions with ease, and certainly not all patients have the willingness to answer them. It sometimes helps if the doctor acknowledges, "I need to ask you some very personal questions and I would like you to answer them as best you can." Either doctor or patient may return to a question from the history that was troublesome on a future visit when more trust has been established.

The physical examination is carried out to determine the woman's general state of health. Height, weight, and blood pressure are measured, and a routine urinalysis for presence of sugar or protein is obtained. Heart and lungs are listened to through a stethoscope. With the patient clad in a hospital gown, the doctor then observes the head and neck, palpates the thyroid gland, and observes and palpates the breasts, abdomen, and pelvic area. Unusual or excessive hair distribution patterns on the face may be evidence of increased male hormone levels. The pubic hair pattern, which is normally triangular, may be diamond-shaped, extending upward toward the navel. This is also a clue that male hormone levels may be high. It is important for the doctor to ask the patient if she has problems with excessive facial hair, since in many cases it will not be visible because of the use of depilatories or shaving or plucking. The size of the breasts has as much to do with general body weight and build and heredity as it does with the amount of estrogen a woman has circulating, but in general, normal breast development means the woman is producing adequate estrogens. The doctor may squeeze behind the nipples to see if any exudate or milk can be expressed. There is a condition in which the nonpregnant woman may produce milk due to abnormal prolactin levels. Finally, the doctor should examine the lower extremities for any abnormalities. If the patient is very thin or obese, recent weight loss or gain should be explored. If the patient is extremely lean and athletic, questions about daily workouts may reveal if the stress is excessive enough to cause hormone imbalance.

During the history and the physical, the doctor should also be asking questions about life-style and work habits. Does the woman smoke cigarettes? Does she drink alcohol? Does she use recreational drugs such as marijuana or cocaine? Is she on any special kind of diet (vegetarian or weight reduction, for example)? How much sleep does she get? Is her occupation pleasant or stressful? Are there any obvious health hazards in her workplace? It is an excellent practice to ask the woman if *she* suspects any particular pattern or problem, since she often has evidence that a certain event seemed to trigger a certain unusual response in her body. The careful doctor is like a detective, leaving no stone unturned in the search for clues.

The Pelvic Exam

An essential part of the first visit is the pelvic examination. The patient is still clad in a hospital gown and lies on the examination table with a drape over her midsection. Her feet are placed in stirrups and her hips are moved as close to the end of the table as possible, where the doctor is seated with bright light upon the area. First the doctor inspects the external genitalia: the vulva, the urethral opening, the clitoris, the mons pubis, and the hair distribution pattern. Then the doctor inserts a speculum into the vagina. These come in several sizes and this procedure should not be uncomfortable. With the internal end of the speculum opened wide and with the aid of the light, the doctor is able to inspect the walls of the vagina and the cervix for unusual growths, sores, signs of discharge, or infection. A Pap test may then be obtained by scraping the cervical opening gently with a small instrument. This test checks for cervical cancer. In addition, the doctor may want to culture the sample for other possible infections such as gonorrhea, chlamydia, or ureaplasma. The two latter organisms are extremely difficult to culture and testing for them may be reserved for later in the investigation.

The doctor will then withdraw the speculum and do a bimanual examination. Inserting the index and middle fingers of one hand into the vagina and pressing down on the abdominal wall with the other, the doctor can feel the size, shape, consistency, and position of the uterus, fallopian tubes, and ovaries. This part of the examination will also reveal any abnormal masses or tumors, existence of pelvic pain, and evidence of adhesions if the organs are not somewhat freely mobile. This part of the examination can be uncomfortable, especially if the woman is very tense, or if she does have pelvic pain due to some disease process. It may help if she concentrates on slow abdominal breathing to relax her muscles. Many doctors finish the exam by inserting a finger into the rectum to check the region behind the uterus (the cul-de-sac) and to check the rectum itself for masses and hemorrhoids. This is unpleasant, but brief.

Basal Temperature Chart

After the completion of the history and the physical and pelvic exams, the most important next step is to teach a woman to begin charting her basal temperature. This serves two functions: First it helps pinpoint the phases of the woman's menstrual cycle, which is helpful in scheduling her other tests. Most tests of the woman have to be performed at a precise time in the preovulatory, ovulatory, or postovulatory part of her menstrual cycle. The most important function of the basal temperature chart, after several cycles have been completed, is that it helps establish whether the woman is ovulating and the approximate time of her ovulation.

The technique for charting basal temperature is simple and easily taught. Doctors generally supply the monthly charts or graphs (simple graph paper may also be used) and the patient only needs an oral thermometer. Special thermometers just for basal charting are available which register only the degrees between 96°F and 100°F to show gradients clearly in tenths of degrees. More sophisticated digital basal thermometers are also available which are quicker, give the actual temperature, and don't break as easily as glass thermometers. Both types are available at most pharmacies without a prescription and range in price from $10 to $40.

The term *basal* means the temperature of the body at rest. This can be accurately measured only just after the woman awakens in the morning, before arising, using the bathroom, or any other activity. The first day of the basal chart is the first day of the menstrual cycle. The temperature, to the nearest tenth of a degree, is marked in the proper square in the graph. Any unusual events that might affect body temperature, such as illness, a sleepless night, large intake of alcohol, or late rising, should be noted. As much as possible, the temperature should be taken about the same time every morning. Some women experience increased vaginal secretions near ovulation; others may have a pain in the ovary upon ovulation (*mittleschmertz*). All these findings should be noted. Sexual activity should be noted on the chart by placing an X or a circle at the time it occurred. Figure 4 gives several examples of basal temperature charts. Most women do not have "classic" charts like those in books, but they learn to interpret their own individual patterns after several months of charts have been kept. It cannot be stated too often that the basal temperature chart is a crude tool at best, but it can be very helpful in pinpointing ovulation and in scheduling tests. Once it has served its purpose for this, it should be discontinued, since long-term basal charting can be a terrible strain on both the woman and her husband.

If a woman is experiencing ovulatory cycles, the time from the onset of her menses to just before ovulation is characterized by a low (about 98°F) temperature that fluctuates slightly. At about the time of ovulation, there may be a dip of several tenths of a degree for one day, followed by an immediate rise of about four-tenths of a degree or more. This higher plateau is maintained until just before the next period, when the temperature falls off to the lower level again. The change in temperature at the midcycle is caused by progesterone entering the system in larger amounts. This is slightly heat producing to the body. A normal ovulatory cycle should be *biphasic*, containing two levels. An anovulatory cycle usually has one fluctuating level and is called *monophasic*. Ovulation is thought to occur within a day or two before the rise in temperature. The interval between ovulation and the next menstruation is about 14 days.

The best timing for sexual relations is within the day before or after ovulation occurs. The obvious flaw of the basal temperature chart is that it can tell when ovulation might have occurred only after the fact. This is why several months of charts tend to be helpful in predicting a current cycle. Most doctors recommend that the couple have relations on alternate nights around the anticipated time of ovulation. Since sperm live up to 48 hours, this should cover the fertile time adequately. For example, if the woman had a 28-day cycle, where ovulation might be supposed to occur on day 14, sexual relations could take place on days 11, 13, and 15, or ideally on days 12, 14, and 16. Sexual activity before and after this critical time should be at the frequency and spontaneity the couple enjoy.

BASAL TEMPERATURE CHART

NAME _Elaine Rogers_   ADDRESS _22 Elm Street_   PHONE _629-4107_

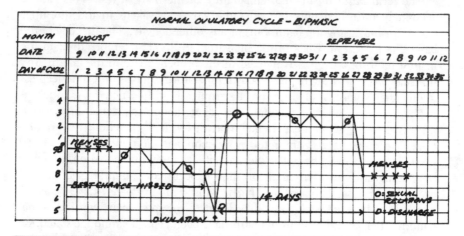

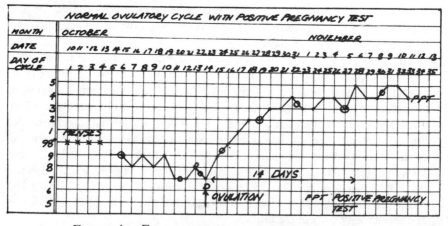

FIGURE 4.   EXAMPLES OF BASAL TEMPERATURE CHARTS

Many couples have difficulty with overfixation on having sexual relations on a specific night. "Sex on demand," as both men and women refer to it, can take all the pleasure out of lovemaking and turn it into an obligation or chore instead. It helps to keep a sense of humor and to keep communications open. If relations do not occur on a given night, it will not be the end of the world. Much more will be said about the feelings about having scheduled sex in the chapter on sexuality.

The basal temperature chart is, incidentally, one of the earliest indicatois of pregnancy. A temperature that stays elevated for 18 to 20 days after ovulation is often indicative of pregnancy. Conversely, the temperature chart that falls off well before the next menstrual cycle may be indicative of a short luteal phase. This can be confirmed through more extensive blood studies.

Blood and Urine Tests

Tests done on the blood and urine of the patient give information about the inner workings of the body. Through the combined use of radioimmunoassays, in which radioactive isotopes are added to blood samples to follow hormonal elements, and ultrasound, which can provide an image of follicular growth, it is now possible to track the entire sequence of a woman's menstrual cycle. Daily tracking would cost a small fortune and is usually not indicated. Generally blood tests are performed at the beginning, middle, and end of the cycle. The tests try to measure the production of the woman's four reproductive hormones: follicular stimulating hormone (FSH), luteinizing hormone (LH), estrogen, and progesterone. The timing of the tests is critical and all should be from the same cycle. The first sample is taken on day 5, 6, or 7 and gives a "baseline" for FSH, LH, and estrogen. The woman returns around the time of ovulation, day 13, 14, or 15, and tests will generally show a higher level of all hormones, including the LH "surge." The final sample is taken anywhere from day 20 to 24 of the cycle. At this time progesterone is measured and should be at its maximum level as estrogen falls off. Presence of male hormones in the woman may indicate polycystic ovarian disease (PCO).

Another blood study screens for the level of prolactin in the woman. This hormone is usually present only after childbirth when it stimulates the milk glands of the breasts to produce milk and inhibits ovulation. Excess prolactin at any other time is abnormal and may indicate the presence of a small tumor of the pituitary. Skull X rays are ordered if a tumor is suspected. Depending on the size, these tumors may be treated by surgical removal or drugs. Thyroid levels should be checked in any patients with symptoms of under- or overactive thyroid.

Studies on the urine are done less frequently since the advent of the sophisticated blood studies. All patients should be checked for presence of protein or sugar in the urine, as well as presence of infections that may indicate other underlying health problems. An exciting innovation in recent years has been urine-testing kits which patients may purchase without prescription to monitor their own urine for the LH surge which generally precedes ovulation by 24 hours. These, in conjunction with the basal temperature chart may help a couple pinpoint ovulation and allow them to time sexual relations or inseminations much more accurately. These kits work in a variety of ways and range in price from $20 up. It is important to read the instructions carefully. If you are taking the drug clomiphene, at least 2 days should elapse before testing or you may get a false reading.

The Postcoital Test

Cervical mucus should undergo changes as ovulation time approaches. The mucus changes from a thick, viscous secretion, impassable to sperm (and most infections), to a crystal-clear, watery secretion. At the optimal time for sperm penetration, it can characteristically be drawn into long elastic threads (called the *spinnbarkeit* phenomenon). Many women monitor their own mucus throughout the cycle and can tell when conditions are optimal for conception. An important early test of the couple's fertility is the postcoital test (also called Hühner test or PK test). The couple are asked to have intercourse on the day of expected ovulation (or a day either way) and to be at the doctor's office within a specified number of hours (from 2 to 8 is common). The woman should not douche or bathe after intercourse. Upon arrival at the doctor's office, the woman is positioned as for a pelvic exam. A sample of her cervical mucus is aspirated from the cervical opening. Examination under the microscope tells the quality and consistency of the mucus and the number and activity of sperm cells. A good postcoital should show abundant, elastic mucus with good numbers of sperm actively swimming in it. The postcoital demonstrates how sperm interact with the vaginal and cervical environment of the woman. A poor result would be recorded if the mucus is thick and impassable or if sperm are found clumped and immobile. This might also indicate a sperm antibody problem. The worst finding is no sperm cells at all, which may indicate azoospermia or a problem in sexual technique. Most often a postcoital is repeated if findings are not good, since the timing may have been the whole problem.

The postcoital should never be used as a replacement for routine semen analysis, since it does not yield much of the valuable information needed. Only in cases of male refusal to participate in semen analysis is the postcoital at least a possible way to check for sperm cells and motility. It should be mentioned that, because the postcoital is a "sex on demand" procedure, the inability of the couple to perform is not uncommon. Some doctors have said it is the most commonly rescheduled test.

Endometrial Biopsy

A biopsy of the lining of the uterus (called endometrium) may be performed at any time after the presumed day of ovulation. If ovulation has occurred, the tissue of the endometrium will reflect the influence of progesterone. If ovulation has not occurred, the tissue will reflect the influence of estrogen, or, occasionally, the lack of any hormonal influence. By looking at the type of tissue obtained and the presumed number of days after ovulation, it is possible to tell whether the woman is producing the appropriate hormones to that phase of her cycle.

Usually the endometrial biopsy is scheduled for the last week in the cycle. The woman has this in the doctor's office, generally without any anesthesia. The woman is positioned as for a pelvic exam. A small instrument is introduced into the cervical opening to gently dilate it. This may cause a cramping sensation. Then a small instrument is introduced into the uterus which scrapes a few small pieces of endometrium. This may also cause cramps and brief discomfort. The tissue is then sent to the pathology laboratory where the specimen is examined microscopically for evidence of progesterone influence. To best interpret the tissue, the doctor must know when the women's next period begins and count back to "tissue date" the specimen. For example a day 25 specimen will have one look, a day 21 specimen, another. When the biopsy shows more than a 2-day lag, it may indicate an inadequate luteal phase.

Some doctors suggest that a couple practice birth control in the endometrial biopsy cycle, although it is unlikely that a pregnancy, had one begun, would be dislodged by the small scraping involved. An early pregnancy test can also be administered the day before the test to rule out pregnancy. This test is often repeated at least twice, since it may show varying results. Many women like to be accompanied by their husbands or a friend for comfort. Afterward a woman may experience a little spotting and continued cramping for a short while.

Hysterosalpingogram

The hysterosalpingogram has replaced the old-fashioned Rubin's test in most practices to provide some information about whether or not the fallopian tubes are patent (open). It may be scheduled as an outpatient test, and since it is an X-ray study, must therefore be done in the X-ray department. Many specialists now combine hysterosalpingogram with laparoscopy, thereby having direct visualization of whether the colored dye flows from the end of the tubes and sparing the patient the discomfort of being awake and without anesthesia for this test.

The timing of this test should always be in the preovulatory phase of the cycle. The woman is positioned in the now familiar pelvic exam position, and her cervix is gently dilated with an instrument. About 3 tablespoons of clear radiopaque dye is injected into the uterus slowly. Cramping will occur as soon as the uterus fills and the sensitive doctor paces the injection to the patient's tolerance and level of discomfort. Fluoroscopy is used while the study is in progress, showing a "real time" image, and several X rays are also taken, from several positions, to get a permanent record of the flow of the dye. Normally the dye fills the uterine cavity, then spills into both fallopian tubes and finally out the ends, where it pools in the peritoneal cavity and is absorbed in time. The contour of the uterine cavity can be seen, and if the dye does not pass through the tubes, a blockage may be revealed. Since temporary spasms due to cramping are also possible, the test must be done slowly and carefully. When the test is done while the patient is under anesthesia during laparoscopy, the doctor is simply looking for the blue dye to appear at the ends of both tubes. If it does not, the X-ray machine can be swung over the patient and the location of the blockage pinpointed on X ray.

This test is among the most uncomfortable the woman must endure. Some doctors premedicate the patient with a nonsteroidal anti-inflammatory drug such as Advil to cut down the pain. Some also recommend use of antibiotics to prevent infection. If laparoscopy is going to be performed anyway, the woman might try to persuade her doctor to do the test then. Otherwise, she should certainly bring her husband or a friend with her and be prepared for cramping and spotting after the test for several hours. She should plan to rest afterward and not return directly to work, if possible.

Ultrasound

One of the exciting diagnostic tools of the last decade has been the ultrasound. In this test, high-frequency sound waves are sent out by a scanning device and transmitted to a small crystal placed on the surface of the body. The sound waves enter the body and echo back when they strike the surface of an organ. The echoes are converted into electrical signals and transferred to a videoscreen, where internal organs are outlined in detail. The images of the videoscreen can be photographed for a permanent record. Sound waves are not related to X rays and carry no risk to the patient. They are routinely done on pregnant women and are not harmful to the developing fetus.

Ultrasound is also completely painless, with one minor exception. In order to have the best possible picture of the pelvic area, the woman is asked to drink volumes of water to fill her bladder completely. The reason is that sound waves are best conducted through water. Fortunately the test takes only a few minutes and the woman is not uncomfortable for long. Ultrasound can reveal the placement of the internal organs and tumors or cysts on the walls of the uterus or ovaries. It has even been refined to the point of being able to count maturing follicles on an ovary and is useful in all procedures that rely upon accurate harvesting of ova or in determining if multiple follicles have been stimulated with the use of certain ovulation induction drugs. If ultrasound has not been indicated before the woman is scheduled for laparoscopy, it is often the first test done when the patient is admitted for her overnight stay in the hospital. Ultrasound done just before laparoscopy gives a doctor a working blueprint. If the patient is going on to laparoscopy, she is then given a light sedative followed by an intravenous injection to make her sleep under short-term anesthesia. A catheter is placed in the bladder to drain the urine and the remaining tests are performed.

Hysteroscopy

With doctors who have expertise in hysteroscopy, this procedure generally precedes laparoscopy and is done under the same anesthesia. This test allows direct visualization of the inside of the uterus through a small scope with fiber-optic light inserted through the cervix. Since the uterine cavity is flat under normal conditions, a clear medium, such as Dextran, is injected to allow the scope a better view. It will reveal abnormal septums, fibroids, polyps, or adhesions. This can be especially important if the woman has used an IUD or had abortions or has a history of infections. Some doctors take advantage of the test to scrape a bit of endometrial tissue for a repeat endometrial biopsy. Some doctors are actually able to cut adhesions, remove small fibroids and polyps, and take care of septum problems viewed through the hysteroscope. This test can also be performed in a doctor's office using a sedative and local anesthetic, but it is quite uncomfortable. Some doctors do not feel the hysteroscopy is necessary.

Laparoscopy

All of the "endoscopic" tests possible on a patient were greatly helped by the discovery of fiber-optic light. This allows a cool, external light to be introduced into the body in the form of a scope and this light will bend around organs and give excellent illumination of the entire peritoneal cavity. While most endoscopic tests enter a natural opening of the body (proctoscope, the rectum; gastroenteroscope, the mouth), the laparoscopy requires a small incision to be made for its entry into the peritoneal cavity. This small incision is usually made next to the navel and can be covered by a Band-Aid at the end, thus giving rise to the terms *belly button surgery* or *Band-Aid operation*.

First it is important to explain that the person doing the laparoscopy is the best qualified person to carry out subsequent surgery on the pelvic organs or tubes, should this be required. While photos can be taken during the procedure, they generally are not, and the view down the scope is only as good as the doctor performing the test. Many doctors will refuse to operate on another's findings, either because they question their expertise, or because they feel the test is too subjective to rely upon another's findings. The patient is well advised to be having laparoscopy only under the hands of a doctor capable enough to do her surgery—including microsurgery and laser surgery—should this be necessary.

Once the patient is placed under short-term anesthesia, a small incision is made beside the navel. A hollow needle is inserted into the cavity and the area is inflated with carbon dioxide gas to raise the abdominal wall and give more space for viewing and maneuvering. The laparoscope is then inserted and the doctor is able to view directly the external wall of the uterus, the outside of the fallopian tubes, and the ovaries. Patches of endometriosis will show up clearly, as will adhesions, clubbing or closure of the fimbriated ends of the tubes, and abnormalities of the ovaries. Some doctors make a second small incision lower down by the pubic hair line so they can introduce a second instrument and have more ability to probe and maneuver. This also allows limited laser surgery or additional diagnostic work such as taking small samples. If dye is going to be injected through the tubes (see hysterosalpingogram), it is done at the end of the procedure. The blue dye can actually be seen as it spills out of the tubes, if they are open.

The woman generally stays overnight in the hospital after laparoscopy and is discharged the next day. She will have a small dressing or Band-Aid over each incision, under which are several stitches. She will often feel sore and the abdominal area will "ache" because of all the manipulation of her organs. This subsides after a day or two. If possible, at least 1 or 2 days of rest at home is a good idea before returning to normal activities. As with many procedures, the range of discomfort and time needed to recover varies widely.

Genetic Counseling

Genetic evaluation of the woman is not carried out routinely, only if there is an indication of a need for it. If there is a family history of genetic disorders, if the woman herself appears to carry a disorder, or if there is a history of repeated spontaneous abortions, with or without fetal abnormalities, it is a good idea to have a closer look. The important test in genetic screening is called a *karyotype*. A blood sample is drawn and the white blood cells are grown in a special medium for 7 days. After this a chemical is added that stops cell division. The cells are placed on a slide and crushed to spread out the chromosomes. The chromosome pairs of 100 cells are counted to determine the chromosomal constitution of the person. If a problem is found, genetic counseling will help the patient and her husband to recognize the risks and the options they face in trying to have a family.

INVESTIGATION OF THE MAN

Until recently, diagnosis and treatment of male infertility fell to the specialty of urology because of the common organs involved. When you realize that urology is the study of the urinary system, you can understand why male infertility was poorly managed and is still decades behind the knowledge of female infertility. In 1976 the American Society of Andrology was formed specifically to study male endocrinology of reproduction and infertility. Reproductive endocrinologists are also playing a major role in diagnosis and medical management of the male, since the male and female have a remarkably similar endocrine mechanism. Surgery of the male is appropriately referred to urologists with special expertise in infertility.

Male fertility may be impaired in any of four ways, and diagnostic tests are aimed at discovering which:

1. There may be a problem with sperm production (spermatogenesis) or in the maturation of sperm.
2. There may be a problem with the ability of sperm to swim (motility).
3. There may be a problem with blockage somewhere in the reproductive tract between where sperm are produced and where they are ejaculated.
4. There may be a problem in depositing the seminal fluid within the vagina.

History and Physical

The history taken from the man, as with the woman, should be a time for establishing rapport and communication with the doctor. Because some of the questions are personal and sensitive in nature, the doctor generally advances from the man's general health and life-style habits to the specifics. It is imperative that history taking allow time separate from the wife so that "secrets" may be revealed if they are relevant to the case.

The doctor will ask about the man's general state of health and any significant diseases or surgeries. Of particular relevance are mumps after the age of puberty, hernia repairs, or history of undescended testicles. The doctor will want to know the approximate age of puberty, when the man became sexually active, and the history of his sexually active years. Has he had many partners? Has he ever contracted a sexually transmitted disease? Has he ever had problems in obtaining erection or achieving orgasm? Has he ever impregnated another woman? Then the history will turn to the current relationship. How long have he and the woman been sexual partners? Have they been exclusive of other partners? Have there been any problems with erection, orgasm, or general satisfaction? Have they ever had a shared infection? What is their usual frequency of intercourse and preferred position(s) and do they use any type of lubricants?

After the sexual history, the doctor will want to know what type of work the man does. A number of occupations are associated with risk of reduced fertility, either because they involve excessive heat or toxins in the workplace. The male is much more at risk than the female is to such risks because he is constantly producing sperm cells, while she has her complete number of ova at birth. The man is also more likely to be influenced by high stress levels for the same reason. The doctor will ask about the man's usual diet and any medications he might be taking. History taking should include any use of alcohol, cigarettes, and "recreational drugs" such as marijuana and cocaine. Extreme exercise regimens may also influence fertility.

The physical exam of the man, while he is dressed in a hospital gown, begins with taking his height, weight, and blood pressure and then doing a routine urinalysis. The doctor observes his general status (nervous, relaxed, robust, thin) and then listens to the heart and lungs, palpates the neck and thyroid, examines the chest and abdomen, and observes the general hair distribution pattern of the pubic area. Usually men have a diamond-shaped hair pattern extending upward toward the navel. The amount of body hair is generally familial and not related to male hormones. The genital area is of most direct concern in the physical exam. The doctor will check the penis for any abnormalities. Then the doctor compresses the scrotum between thumb and palm, using the fingers to distinguish each testicle, the epididymis coiled on top of it, and the vas deferens, which runs like a cord up the back of each testicle. Some doctors measure the testes with calipers; others only note the general size. If a man has never been taught to check his testicles for cancer, this is an excellent time to learn. (Cancer of the testicles is the leading cancer in men between twenty-five to thirty-five years of age. Early detection offers an excellent chance of survival.)

Examination for Varicocele

Varicocele is thought by many specialists to be a leading cause of infertility in men. It can generally be palpated in the physical exam. It is most commonly found on the left side and is a bundle of dilated veins similar to varicose veins. It also may sometimes occur on the right or on both sides. The doctor asks the man to stand up, hold his breath, and bear down hard. This will push blood into the varicocele and make it easier to feel. A small varicocele may cause infertility as well as a large one and may elude the physical exam. The Doppler stethoscope, an ultrasound stethoscope magnifier used by obstetricians to hear fetal heartbeats, can help in locating a varicocele. As the patient bears down, the doctor will hear abnormal blood sounds where the spermatic cord and its artery pump blood into the testicle. A new thermogram technique is also being used to locate varicoceles. If one testicle registers warmer than the other, a varicocele is likely present. Not all varicoceles require surgical correction. If the semen analysis shows a highly stressed sperm pattern, it is likely that surgery will help. It should be noted that not all doctors believe varicoceles to be a cause of infertility, especially if the semen analysis is normal.

Prostate Examination

The patient is now asked to bend over and the doctor inserts one finger in the rectum to feel the prostate gland. If the gland is tender or seems infected, the doctor will massage it to try to express a little fluid through the penis for culture of organisms and presence of white blood cells. This is uncomfortable but only lasts a moment.

The Semen Analysis

Without any question, the single most important test of the male is the semen analysis. Also called a "sperm count," the test in fact measures many other important factors: the number of million sperm per cubic centimeter (cc), the ability of the sperm to swim (motility), the size and shape of the sperm cells (morphology), the total semen volume, the viscosity or liquefaction of the ejaculate, the presence of seminal fructose, cultures for infectious organisms, and presence of sperm antibodies. The results gained from a semen analysis will be only as good as the expertise of the lab doing the work and, they also depend upon proper collection and timely delivery to the lab.

Collection of the specimen can be done in several ways. From the doctor's point of view, the best way is to have the man produce the specimen right at the lab so it can be analyzed immediately. This is the only way to see the change from the coagulated state of the ejaculate to the liquefied state some 20 to 30 minutes later. The man is asked to masturbate a specimen into a clean glass container in a private room near the lab. Many men simply cannot do this, and the understanding doctor allows that a specimen produced at home and brought right in (being kept warm if it is cold weather) is almost as good and much more comfortable for most men. The specimen should be delivered within 1 to 2 hours. Some men are unable to masturbate either through their own convictions or dictates of their religion. In such cases, a nonspermicidal condom may be worn and regular intercourse may occur. If there is a religious proscription against birth control as well, a small pinhole can be made in the condom, about halfway down, which usually satisfies this problem. The entire contents of the condom are emptied into a glass jar and brought to the lab. This is less desirable because there will be bacteria from the penis in the sample and some of the semen lost in the condom. The least desirable collection technique is coitus interruptus, because it is virtually impossible to catch the first few droplets of semen which contain many of the sperm. However, *any* collection technique is preferable to none. If a man refuses to submit a semen specimen, the postcoital test is a last resort which gives some indication if there are any sperm cells and what their activity is.

Because the man is not cyclic, he can produce his specimen at any time. There does not need to be any "saving up" sperm for the test. In fact, the interval between normal sexual relations makes the most sense, since it shows what the man is actually delivering into the woman. If the couple has relations more than every other night, abstinence for 24 hours before the test is advised. The semen analysis should be done as early in the couple's investigation as possible, since a problem found in the man should be corrected before the woman is subjected to all her tests. It is common for the semen analysis to be repeated at least once, since fertility fluctuates. If the investigation of the woman is very lengthy, it is a good idea to have the man's fertility rechecked periodically.

If a semen analysis is normal, the results will reflect the following:

Sperm count. The range of "normal" for the number of million sperm per cc was 50 to 60 for many years. Counts below 10 million are considered poor, but recent studies show that counts of 20 million or more are considered fertile if all other factors are favorable. In general, the higher the sperm count, the better the chances of conception, but excessively high sperm counts may be characterized by poor motility and may actually be a deterrent.

Motility. Some specialists feel that motility is the single most important factor in the fertility of the male. Two aspects of motility need to be evaluated: (1) the number of active cells as a percentage of the total cells, and (2) the quality of the movement of the cells. The first level is measured in a percentage from 0 to 100. Two or three hours after ejaculation, 50 percent of the sperm cells should be active; more is even better. The progression of sperm cells in a straight line across a grid is rated from 0 (no progression) to 4 (excellent progression). A score of 2 or better is satisfactory.

Morphology. Sperm cells are not all alike. There are immature forms, abnormal forms, and amorphous cells in any ejaculate. In a normal ejaculate, at least 60 percent of cells should be normal forms. Evidence of large numbers of immature cells, called *spermatids*, or presence of tapering forms may be evidence of a varicocele.

Total volume. The usual semen specimen falls between 2 and 5 cc of ejaculate. Abnormally high or low volumes may be a fertility problem.

Liquefaction. Human semen is ejaculated in a liquid state. It immediately coagulates into a pearly gel and then liquefies again within 20 to 30 minutes. Failure to liquefy may impede motility of sperm. *Viscosity* is the consistency of the semen after liquefaction has occurred. High viscosity may be a factor in poor motility.

Seminal fructose. If the specimen is devoid of sperm, the doctor may test the semen for seminal fructose, which is normally produced in the seminal vesicles. If it is present, blockage somewhere below the seminal vesicles is suspected. If it is absent, congenital absence of the vas deferens or seminal vesicles is likely. This can be confirmed by X-ray studies.

Cultures. The doctor will usually culture the semen for presence of chlamydia, ureaplasma, and any other bacteria noted in the specimen.

Sperm antibodies. An area that is still hotly contested as to its very existence as well as its significance in fertility is presence of antibodies against sperm in the semen specimen. If large numbers of sperm are found clumped together in clusters, the specimen may be tested for antibodies. First sperm are separated from seminal fluid and placed in a neutral fluid. If they do well in the neutral fluid, the sperm themselves appear free of antibodies. Then sperm known to be free of antibodies are mixed with the semen. If they clump, it is assumed the semen is defective.

Other tests. A normal semen analysis still may not confirm that a man is fertile. Researchers are constantly looking for new and better tests. One recent test, considered controversial by many, is the ability of human sperm to penetrate a specially prepared hamster egg. Some feel that inability to penetrate an ovum may be an infertility problem when a "normal" male is not able to impregnate a "normal" female.

Blood Studies

Unlike the woman, the man may be tested on any day with one blood sample to show his hormone levels. Radioimmunoassay of blood tests for FSH, LH, and testosterone levels. It is interesting to most couples that the messengers sent out from the pituitary are virtually identical in male and female—FSH and LH are actually named for the actions they produce in the female, but the same hormones are present in the male. The target organ, of course, is very different, being the ovaries in the woman and the testicles in the man.

If blood tests show low FSH and LH levels, the problem lies somewhere in the hypothalmic-pituitary centers. If blood tests show high FSH and LH levels, the problem probably lies in the testicles. Sperm production has two separate systems: Leydig's cells are in charge of producing testosterone; spermatogonia are in charge of sperm production. If the FSH is high, the spermatogonia are in question; if the LH is high, the Leydig's cells are at fault. If both hormones are high, neither system is working properly. If all hormones are normal, yet a man has a low sperm count, there may be a problem in the transport system. This requires surgical tests.

Testicular Biopsy and Vasogram

A biopsy of the testicle provides a blueprint of the sperm production factory. The vasogram, usually done at the same time, is an X-ray dye study which outlines the sperm transport system and reveals any obstructions. Both are usually done in "same-day surgery" with the man under short-term anesthetic. The scrotum is opened with a small incision and the doctor locates the lower end of the vas deferens. Radiopaque dye is slowly injected and should reveal all internal passages, from the epididymis, up the vas deferens, into the seminal vesicles and ejaculatory ducts. X rays are taken and if any blockage is present, it will show up.

When the vasogram has been completed, a small wedge of tissue is removed from the testicles for examination. The incision is closed with several stitches and an ice bag applied. Ice and aspirin usually keep the discomfort to a minimum, although the man may wish to wear an athletic supporter for a few days. The biopsy is sent to a lab and examined carefully. If spermatogonia cells are present, sperm cells in all stages of development should be in evidence. If no spermatogonia cells are found, sperm production is hopeless, even though Leydig's cells may produce testosterone. Therapy is based upon what cells are found and what they are capable of producing.

Genetic Counseling

Infertility is rarely caused by an inherited defect, simply because infertile men and women do not bear children. However, analysis of chromosomes may be indicated by some finding in the investigation, or by the characteristics of the man himself. Also, if the family history suggests a history of genetic disorders that might be passed on to children, the couple may want to have a test of their chromosomes.

REFERRAL POINTS IN THE INVESTIGATION

If the couple has not chosen an infertility specialist at the outset, there are some logical points at which the couple should decide to seek this additional expertise. The American Fertility Society has been very cautious in suggesting referral, partly because it is a membership organization open to all doctors, including ob/gyn doctors and specialists. RESOLVE has been more outspoken in recommending a specialist *before* laparoscopy, and in event of any of these findings:

1. In general, the couple should seek a specialist after the postcoital test and before the more sophisticated tests are begun.
2. Patients requiring surgery should seek a specialist.
3. A woman with a history of two or more miscarriages should seek a specialist.
4. Sperm antibody problems, whether in the male or the female (it is often difficult to tell which) should be referred to a specialist.
5. Problems of ovulation requiring ovulation-inducing drugs should be referred to a specialist.
6. Any case of "unexplained infertility" going on more than two years in the face of normal tests should be referred to a specialist.
7. Men with abnormal semen analysis should seek a specialist.

If you make the change to a new doctor, select carefully, using the criteria suggested in chapter 3. You should have your records sent to the new doctor so they will be there for your first visit. You probably will not have to repeat tests if you go early in the investigation. Many of the later tests are so subject to the ability of the doctor that a specialist is not likely to accept a nonspecialist's results.

5. Causes and Treatment of Female Infertility

A *childless housewife* . . .
How tenderly
She touches
Little dolls for sale.

RANSETSU

When a proper investigation of the couple has been conducted by a doctor with expertise in infertility, a known cause is found in about 90 percent of all cases. A problem of the female partner is found in 35 percent of the cases; a problem of the male partner is found in 35 percent as well. In 20 percent of the cases, some problem is found with both partners, often a minor problem but compounded by the fact that there are several elements involved. Finally, about 10 percent of all couples do not get an answer to why they are infertile. These "unexplained infertility" cases are among the hardest for couples to bear and receive special attention in chapter 14.

A woman may be unable to conceive or carry pregnancy for any of the following reasons:

1. There may be a problem with ovulation, or with the endocrine system that influences the menstrual cycle.
2. There may be a mechanical barrier to the union of ovum and sperm.
3. There may be structural or functional problems with the uterus or cervix.

OVULATION AND ENDOCRINE PROBLEMS

In about half of all female infertility, a problem of ovulation or the endocrine system is found to be the cause. The tests that pinpoint the disorders are the BBT, blood studies for FSH, LH, estrogen, and progesterone, thyroid and male hormone levels, and elevated prolactin levels. Fortunately, because of the new drugs recently available, ovulation and endocrine disorders are among the most hopeful for successful treatment. Some practices quote success rates of 75 to 90 percent for specific conditions; others may respond at a lower rate.

Nonfunctional Ovaries

In order for there to be ovulation, functional ovaries must be present. There are several situations when this is not the case. In *Turner's syndrome*, a genetic disorder that occurs rarely, the woman receives a single X instead of an XX sex chromosome. The ovaries fail to develop in these cases. Those women affected do not develop secondary sex characteristics and do not menstruate. The condition cannot be corrected, but those women can obtain normal maturity and menses by receiving estrogen replacement therapy. Sometimes ovarian tissue fails early in adulthood for unknown reasons. *Premature ovarian failure* is frequently preceded by a history of scanty and erratic menstrual periods which were probably anovulatory. This situation is one that can be masked by prolonged use of the birth control pill. It is also a condition that cannot be corrected once it has occurred, but the woman can take estrogen replacement to keep from aging prematurely. *Hyperstimulation* of the ovaries with powerful fertility drugs is a rare situation which may result in loss of ovarian function. Surgical removal of ovaries (*oophorectomy*), with or without a hysterectomy, will result in loss of fertility. A special section in chapter 14 deals with issues of early ovarian/uterine loss. An interesting new technology (donation of ova or embryos) now makes it possible for women with a uterus but without ovarian function to become pregnant. While the procedure is still in the early stages, it offers some hope for this population. See chapter 8 for discussion of this.

Nonspecific Anovulation

About 25 percent of ovulatory problems involve a slight irregularity of the hormonal axis. Called *nonspecific anovulation*, the pattern may be one of perfectly normal periods for a few months, followed by several months that appear anovulatory. Remember that just because a woman menstruates does not prove she has ovulated. Some women ovulate only a few months out of the year. This can be identified by use of basal temperature charts and blood studies to look at the progesterone level. Of all ovulatory problems, these are most easily treated. With use of a drug called clomiphene citrate, the system usually regulates itself within a few cycles. Clomiphene is generally taken days 5 to 9 of the woman's cycle. This is also used for *post-pill anovulation*, where a woman does not regain her menstrual cycle after using the birth control pill.

Polycystic Ovarian Disease

Another common and complex cause of ovulatory failure is polycystic ovarian disease (PCO). It is also known as Stein-Leventhal syndrome after the doctors who identified it in the 1930s. In PCO there are several discernible symptoms: The woman has absent or infrequent periods, she may be obese and have excessive hair growth on the face and breasts, and the ovaries on palpation and observation are enlarged with multiple cysts on them. The reasons for these symptoms are a basic hormonal imbalance of a distinctive pattern: low to low-normal FSH, constant high levels of estrogens, high-pulsating LH levels, low progesterone, and elevated weak male hormone levels. These hormone levels are seen on any day of the month, which is not cyclic. Something is wrong with the hormonal axis between the hypothalamus-pituitary center and the ovaries. No one really knows which area begins the problem, but once it has started it snowballs. Because the follicles never release an egg, they swell and turn into cysts in the ovaries. Cells around these cysts produce excessive amounts of weak male hormones, which are responsible for the excessive hair growth. The weak male hormones are picked up by body fat cells and converted to estrogen. This accounts for the high estrogen level, which in turn inhibits the FSH level and encourages the high LH levels. A major concern with PCO is that the constant high estrogen level overstimulates the lining of the uterus, which does not shed since there is no menstruation. This can encourage abnormal growths and even malignancy. Also, the woman cannot ovulate or become pregnant. She may also consult her doctor because of the troublesome cosmetic side effects of her disease.

Polycystic ovarian disease is often difficult to diagnose, since symptoms may vary from extreme to slight. Usually the tip-offs are very enlarged ovaries (as much as three times normal), basal charts that show continued anovulatory cycles, along with blood studies showing elevated male hormones and a constant estrogen supply. It is difficult to know if the male hormones are being produced by the ovary or by the adrenal gland. To check for this, *a dexamethasone suppression test* is performed. This involves taking a drug to suppress adrenal activity. If the excess male hormones are coming from the adrenals, levels of these hormones (DHEA—sulfate-specific adrenal androgens) will drop. In this case the drug prednisone, a synthetic steroid, will be prescribed and resumption of normal ovulation may occur.

The possibility of *hyperprolactinemia* (elevated prolactin levels) should also be considered, since 30 to 40 percent of patients with PCO have this problem as well. Many doctors feel it is wise to utilize laparoscopy to visualize the ovaries directly and rule out any other fertility problems before starting treatment. Others are now using ultrasound to observe the ovaries.

The immediate goal of treatment is to start menstrual bleeding again to avoid malignancy. This is accomplished by giving progesterone. If pregnancy is also a goal, ovulation must be induced by use of fertility drugs (see pages 48 to 49). Once ovulation occurs, the hormone imbalance and symptoms of PCO usually disappear. If there is no other fertility problem, about 65 percent of the patients go on to become pregnant. Some women with PCO will need ovulation induction each time they want to become pregnant; others remain cured by the treatment. For those who do not wish to become pregnant, artificial menstruation with progesterone at least 4 to 5 times a year will reduce risks of uterine cancer from their high estrogen levels if they are not cycling normally.

Luteal Phase Defects

The luteal phase of the menstrual cycle is the 10 to 14 days after ovulation. Following release of the egg from the ovarian follicle, the corpus luteum forms, which takes over progesterone production and is responsible for producing the lush endometrial tissue of the uterus in preparation for the fertilized egg. Once a fertilized egg implants, HCG from the cells destined to become the placenta tells the corpus luteum to go on producing progesterone to preserve the pregnancy and prevent menstruation until the placenta can take over this function completely at about 12 weeks of gestation.

About 3 to 8 percent of infertile women have a luteal phase defect present. This is due to a low progesterone level caused by poor corpus luteum development and concurrent substandard uterine endometrium to support implantation. Such women often have a history of frequent early miscarriage. Occult pregnancy (miscarriage before pregnancy has been confirmed) may also be occurring. Women more than thirty-five years of age seem to have this problem more than younger women.

Diagnosis is made by study of the BBT and evidence of a luteal phase that is consistently 10 days or less. Blood serum progesterone tests drawn 4 to 11 days prior to menstruation may be low. Endometrial biopsy taken 2 to 3 days before expected menstruation will show a lag of 2 or more days in endometrial development.

Treatment of luteal phase defects depends on the cause. The problem can be a defective LH stimulus from the pituitary, in which case HCG will supply the missing hormone to the ovaries. The problem may be premature death of the corpus luteum itself, in which case vaginal suppositories of natural progesterone are given to the woman. The progesterone is absorbed directly by the endometrium or the bloodstream. These suppositories are continued for 10 to 12 weeks into pregnancy, when the placenta is presumed to have taken over progesterone function. Many women are concerned about taking hormones in pregnancy due to the DES disaster of the recent past. Studies indicate that natural progesterones do not have associated risks. Synthetic forms of progesterone are never prescribed. The main problem with progesterone suppositories is that they are not available at many pharmacies (RESOLVE can supply the names of pharmacies that ship them) and that they are somewhat messy to use. Some doctors are using intermuscular injections of natural progesterone with good results. Luteal phase defects are most successfully diagnosed and treated by infertility specialists, and in their hands patients have an excellent chance of achieving and carrying a pregnancy to term.

Ovulation Induction Drugs

Ovulation induction is accomplished by use of one of several major fertility drugs available since the 1960s. *These drugs are potent and should be used only by an infertility specialist.* Clomiphene citrate is the safest and most commonly used fertility drug. It works by stopping up estrogen receptors in the hypothalamus and tricking the brain into thinking there is no estrogen in the system. A woman begins clomiphene on day 4 of her cycle and usually continues for 5 days. The hypothalamus, sensing no estrogen, calls on the pituitary to increase FSH production. This large dose of FSH reaches the ovaries and stimulates egg production. As egg production develops, estrogen in increasing amounts enters the bloodstream, but the receptors still don't detect it. When clomiphene is stopped after 5 days, the hypothalamus suddenly recognizes a massive level of estrogen. It responds by sending a message to the pituitary to release a large surge of LH to the ovaries. The LH burst "kicks" the egg free from the ovary, and then natural progesterone production will begin by the corpus luteum, which forms from the follicle. Sometimes the LH burst is not sufficient and an injection of *human chorionic gonadotropin* (HCG) is also given to boost the LH level. HCG, which very closely resembles LH, is a chemical derived from the placenta of pregnant women. Clomiphene is relatively safe because it is not introducing hormones into the system (it is an antiestrogen) but rather tricks the body into making more of its own hormones. Because the FSH dose is higher than usual, increased incidence of twins is seen (about 1 in 50, twice the normal rate).

Clomiphene may also cause cervical mucus to be scanty and thick at ovulation, but this can be monitored and treated with a small dose of estrogen given with the clomiphene. This drug works about 75 percent of the time in producing an ovulation.

The big gun in the ovulation induction arsenal is *human menopausal gonadotropin* (also called Pergonal). This drug is an equal combination of LH and FSH obtained from the urine of menopausal women. Menopausal women have excessively high levels of FSH and LH in their systems due to the fact that the ovaries do not respond to shut off these messengers. Where clomiphene works on the hypothalamus, Pergonal bypasses the brain and acts directly on the ovaries, encouraging them to develop eggs. A woman takes Pergonal by injection for 5 to 10 days each month. To avoid hyperstimulation of the ovary or multiple birth (this is the drug that has been responsible for occasional quintuplets) careful daily monitoring of the blood for estrogen level will reflect the degree of stimulation. Ultrasound can also be used to count the number and size of maturing follicles. When it appears that one or two are ready for release, an injection of HCG is given to help the egg(s) release. With careful monitoring, Pergonal is a very effective drug which results in a single birth 80 percent of the time. When gestations are multiple, 75 percent of the time they are twins.

Elevated Prolactin Levels

Normally, prolactin is seen after birth in the nursing mother. It stimulates milk production in the breasts and has an inhibitory action on ovulation. Nonpregnant women who have amenorrhea (absence of menstrual periods) and galactorrhea (milk in the breasts) are suspected of having this problem. Sometimes the woman has had a pregnancy in the past and the prolactin level persists after lactation is stopped. This is called the *Chiari-Fromel syndrome.* Sometimes the cause is a small pituitary tumor, which is called *Forbes-Albright syndrome.* It has been seen in women after use of some psychiatric drugs such as phenothiazines and reserpine. Most commonly it occurs after oral-contraceptive therapy and is called "post-pill" *galactorrhea-amenorrhea* syndrome.

Serum prolactin levels can be measured by radioimmunoassay. Normal levels range from 2 to 15 ng/ml. In galactorrhea-amenorrhea syndrome, levels as high as 100 ng/ml may be seen. In 1978 the Food and Drug Administration approved the drug bromocriptine mesylate for use in patients with elevated prolactin levels. First a skull X ray or CAT scan should be done to rule out pituitary tumors. If one is found, surgical removal may be advised, although, if the tumor is not too large, bromocriptine therapy may control it. Bromocriptine is taken 2 to 3 times a day at a therapeutic dose of about 2.5

mg. Studies have shown that 80 percent of patients will resume normal menses in about 8 weeks and 90 percent will resume normal ovulation. Side effects are mild and the drug appears low in risk, although doctors generally advise the patient to use a barrier method of birth control while on the drug and that pregnancy be attempted only after normal menses have resumed and the drug is stopped. The problem is that bromocriptine is a treatment but not a cure for the problem, and if treatment is stopped for a length of time, amenorrhea will return. A number of women have conceived while on bromocriptine and their rate of birth defects does not exceed that of the normal population. Women who do conceive while on the medication stop taking it and are instructed to avoid breast-feeding after delivery, since this may increase their prolactin production.

Other uses for bromocriptine are being reported. Use in luteal phase defects associated with high prolactin levels is successful. Also use in men with high prolactin levels is promising.

Other Endocrine Problems

Any type of thyroid problem should be cleared up before the doctor attempts to regulate or treat a problem of ovulation. If blood levels show an underactive thyroid, synthetic thyroid hormones will increase production. If the thyroid is overactive, suppressive drugs are given. An underactive thyroid can be responsible for an excess of prolactin in some cases. Thyroid stimulating hormone (TSH), working overtime to drive an impaired gland, may also stimulate the cells that make prolactin.

MECHANICAL BARRIERS TO CONCEPTION

Obstructions in the reproductive tract account for almost 40 percent of female infertility problems. There are several major causes: pelvic inflammatory disease caused by sexually transmitted disease or by infection introduced through an IUD, instrumentation, or infection from within; endometriosis; and postpartum or postsurgical adhesions and scarring. Each of these will be discussed.

Pelvic Inflammatory Disease

Each year more than a million women are treated for pelvic inflammatory disease (PID). This disease can be life-threatening in its full-blown stages and especially has a devastating effect upon the reproductive organs. Almost all pelvic infections are caused by organisms introduced via sexual intercourse. A woman who has had one episode of PID has a 15 percent risk of infertility; after two infections, there is a 50 percent risk; after three infections, risk of infertility climbs to almost 75 percent.* Twenty years ago blocked tubes, pelvic adhesions, and scarring accounted for about 25 percent of female infertility. Today that figure has almost doubled and is due in part to the skyrocketing number of pelvic infections. Not only are young women sexually active with multiple partners at younger ages, the number and nature of infectious agents transmitted sexually has changed.

Any bacteria can cause PID under the right circumstances. The most common and most dangerous invaders are gonorrhea, streptococcus, chlamydia, and ureaplasma. Gonorrheal bacteria excrete endotoxins inside their cell walls. When the walls rupture, the toxins pour out. The bacteria may travel into the fallopian tubes and rupture, causing the endotoxins to dissolve the tube's lining. The tube collapses and its walls stick together and the end fills with excretions (called *hydrosalpinx*). The ends of the tubes can seal shut. Streptococcal bacteria excrete exotoxins through their cell walls. These tunnel their way directly through muscle and tissue. The dead tissue left behind is ripe for invasion by anaerobes (organisms that grow only in absence of oxygen).

The most dangerous sexually transmitted disease today is a newly recognized organism called chlamydia. This little-known and often misdiagnosed infection now surpasses gonorrhea as the leading sexually transmitted disease in America. Chlamydia is by definition a bacterium, but it closely resembles a large virus. Like a virus, chlamydia lives and multiplies inside other cells. When the host cells eventually fill up and explode, the bacteria escape to invade new cells. Because the organism prefers to invade epithelial (lining) cells, the inside of the fallopian tubes is an ideal target. Research and diagnosis of chlamydia has been hampered by the fact that it is so fragile an organism. It breaks down readily when removed from its territory. Until several years ago, the only way to test for chlamydia was to grow cultures in a difficult, time-consuming, and expensive procedure available at only a few hundred laboratories in the country. New tests now available nationwide do not require cultures and can be done quickly and inexpensively by any laboratory. The worst problem with chlamydia is that it is a relatively "silent" infection, which can do great damage before symptoms are present. Symptoms, if they do occur, include thick yellow discharge from the vagina, painful urination, and eventually fever and pelvic pain. Men notice symptoms such as painful urination and urethral discharge more commonly than do women. These symptoms are often mistaken for gonorrhea or even urinary

---

* Joseph H. Bellina, M.D., and Josleen Wilson, *You Can Have a Baby* (New York: Crown Publishers, 1985), p. 235.

tract infections. As a result, misdiagnosis is common and treatment with penicillin (for gonorrhea) is ineffective. The medication that does treat chlamydia is tetracycline, which should be taken for 7 or more days. Both partners must be treated! Pregnant women with chlamydia will infect their babies at birth and should take erythromycin. Studies have shown that a single attack of chlamydia is three times as likely to cause sterility in women than is gonorrhea. Chlamydia has been called an "epidemic" in recent years. As many as one third of all PID cases are now caused by this organism.

Ureaplasma is still an enigma as to how it causes infertility and even *whether* it causes infertility. Women who have cultured positive for the organism and been treated often become pregnant. There are two types of ureaplasma: U. urealyticum and mycoplasma. The latter is often found in tiny colonies in a variety known as *T-mycoplasma*. Either type may be associated with infertility. Although ureaplasma is associated with PID, it is not known if it is an infection per se or simply changes the body's defense mechanism against other organisms. There are no symptoms with ureaplasma infections. They are usually picked up when other cultures are performed. Culturing for ureaplasma requires a cervical or urethral swab from the woman and a urethral swab from her partner. Cultures grow only on a special, delicate medium, which must be kept frozen, defrosted to receive the culture, and then shipped frozen again to a laboratory. Treatment of ureaplasma is a 10-day course of tetracycline, after which 90 percent of the cases appear cured. Both partners must be treated! Ureaplasma may also be implicated in miscarriage and stillbirth, as it has been cultured from aborted fetuses. More research needs to be done to understand how ureaplasma causes infertility and how it can be more readily detected and treated.

Viral infections that can be sexually transmitted include herpes simplex, condyloma acuminata (venereal warts), and the virus associated with AIDS (acquired immune deficiency syndrome). Unlike bacteria, they do not directly invade the reproductive tract to cause mechanical obstructions, but they may lead the way for other infections by breaking down cervical mucus. Viral infections also change the milieu of the vagina, which may become hostile to sperm. AIDS is of concern, not because it causes infertility, but because it is a lethal disease for which treatment has not yet been found.

Not all pelvic infections are sexually transmitted. There can also be invasion from within the body. Ruptured appendix is a leading cause of scarring and damage to the pelvic cavity of the female. Tuberculosis, in countries where it is still prevelant, may invade the pelvic area after migrating from the lungs and forming abscesses. Pelvic tuberculosis causes profound scarring and adhesions which makes reconstructive surgery almost impossible.

It is thought that bacteria are able to attach themselves to sperm and use this form of transport to reach the fallopian tubes and pelvic cavity. Teenage girls are known to have a longer estrogen phase in their menstrual cycle than adult women, are making them more vulnerable to sperm penetration of the cervical mucus (as much as 3 to 5 days longer). Contraceptives, if they are used, may affect the risk of PID one way or another. Barrier methods such as the condom or diaphragm block entry completely. The birth control pill creates a tough cervical mucus all month and is thought to help block sperm penetration. However, some evidence reveals that chlamydia is *more* common in women using the Pill. The IUD makes a woman who has never borne children 7 to 10 times more susceptible to develop PID.

Before surgical attempts can be made to reconstruct damaged reproductive organs, a diagnosis of the organism(s) involved and treatment with the proper antibiotic is necessary. The sooner the diagnosis and treatment are initiated, the less the damage to correct. Patients with mild symptoms are treated with the proper antibiotic and watched closely. If the symptoms do not subside in 24 to 48 hours, the patient may be admitted to the hospital for intravenous antibiotic therapy. In some cases the doctor starts a broad spectrum drug such as doxycycline before the results of cultures are known to save time and prevent further damage to organs. Women with moderate to severe symptoms are always admitted to the hospital and started on an intravenous therapy at once. Laparoscopy may be used to give the doctor direct visualization of the area and a chance to aspirate fluid samples and make cultures from a variety of locations. In cases of rampant infections, usually involving a combination of bacteria, the situation may be life threatening. The reproductive organs may be so diseased that total hysterectomy/oophorectomy must be performed. While this is rare and extreme, it is generally presumed that fertility was lost even before surgery took place.

Endometriosis

The second leading cause of mechanical obstruction in women is a condition called *endometriosis*. About 15 percent of all women have endometriosis, and about 50 percent of those experience infertility. Although it can occur at any age after puberty, it is most often seen in women thirty to forty years of age who have not borne children. It is thought that endometriosis occurs because normal endometrial lining of the uterus escapes out the fallopian tubes and into the pelvic cavity, possibly at the time of menstruation. These cells then implant and grow where they lodge, in the tubes, on the ovaries, in the peritoneal cavity, and even on the outside of the bowel and bladder. The endometrial tissue reacts to the hormonal cycle just as uterine lining does, building up under the influence of estrogen and progesterone, and sloughing off when menstruation begins. In these locations, unlike in the uterus, the menstrual flow has no place to exit the body. The area around the implants becomes inflamed and scar tissue may develop. In more serious cases, bands of scar tissue called adhesions may develop that displace or "freeze" the organs in the pelvis so they cannot move. Endometrial implants may also rupture and seed new implants to other areas, thus aggravating the condition. In addition to creating mechanical obstructions to conception, mild endometriosis, it is theorized, may cause some kind of autoimmune reaction because the misplaced implants are viewed as "foreign cells" to the body, which sends out antibodies that kill sperm or the fertilized egg. Another theory is based on the fact that there appears to be a higher level of prostaglandin in women with endometriosis, which may play a role in increased early pregnancy loss. A final theory is that endometriosis can shorten the luteal phase of the cycle. Whatever the mechanism, endometriosis can be a distressing and debilitating cause of infertility.

The major symptom of endometriosis is severe pain and cramping just before, during, and after menstruation. This can be incapacitating to some women. The pain is caused by the swelling and bleeding of the implants in nonuterine areas, and subsequent inflammation and scar tissue development. Pain during intercourse is also a frequent symptom, especially if implants are located in the "cul-de-sac" area behind the uterus or the organs are bound down with adhesions. Even though endometriosis is a disease seen in older women, it may have been present for years, causing painful periods. Doctors used to pat women on the head and tell them that menstrual discomfort was normal and a small price to pay for eventual motherhood. Endometriosis tends to run in families, and it was often the mother who told her daughter that childbearing would cause the pain to go away one day. Indeed, pregnancy does put endometriosis to rest for nine months, since menstruation is not taking place. But it does not "cure" most situations.

Diagnosis of endometriosis is made by several means. Often her history and physical and pelvic exams suggest to the doctor that a woman is suffering from this disease. Laparoscopy will confirm this and will tell the extent of the damage and which course of therapy makes the most sense. No other laboratory studies or tests will diagnose this problem. BBT charts will often be normal. In women with mild forms of endometriosis, only laparoscopy will discover it. Endometriosis is classified from Stage I (minimal disease) to Stage II (mild disease) to Stage III (moderate disease) and Stage IV (extensive disease).

Treatment of endometriosis is controversial and divided between advocates of surgical intervention to "clean out" the implants and free up adhesions and advocates of a course of medical therapy first, usually with the drug danazol to let the body repair itself if it can. Most doctors use a combination of these treatments in one order or the other. For Stage I or II endometriosis, a doctor may prescribe danazol first. Danazol is a synthetic weak male hormone that stops ovulation by creating a "pseudomenopause" state. Without hormonal stimulation, endometrial implants do not grow; in fact they shrink and disappear after a few months. A small number of women experience side effects such as weight gain, facial hair growth, or acne, but these reverse when the drug is stopped after three to six months. Ovulation will return spontaneously within 6 weeks. After medical treatment of Stage I and II, 60 to 70 percent of women will achieve pregnancy Treatment for Stages III or IV have to consider the woman's age. If the woman is under thirty-five, a nine-month course of danazol will be tried, followed by second-look laparoscopy. Microsurgery or laser surgery (discussed more fully below) can be used to clean up the remaining disease. Some doctors then follow up surgery with another course of three months of danazol. If the woman is over thirty-five, time is of the essence and surgery may be done immediately and followed by three months of danazol. Success rates with new surgical techniques and danazol approach the same as for medical management of Stages I and II. If the woman does become pregnant, she is at increased risk of ectopic pregnancy (pregnancy in the tube) and this should be monitored via blood levels and ultrasound. An important point to make about endometriosis is that it cannot be "cured." Treatment only holds the disease in check and, hopefully, allows the woman to have her family.

Sometimes the pain caused by endometriosis is so incapacitating that the doctor will perform a presacral neurectomy, cutting certain nerves that transmit the pain messages. If a woman is through having children, or does not wish to have children, severe cases may be more successfully treated by total hysterectomy and removal of ovaries. Since this is a major decision, a woman should get a second or even third opinion on the risks and benefits involved.

Microsurgery and Laser Surgery for Obstructions

The advent of microsurgery (operating under magnifying lenses) has changed many types of surgical procedures in the past few decades. Beginning in surgery on the eye and tiny blood vessels, microsurgery became clearly beneficial to other areas as well. Some specialists now believe *only* microsurgery should be performed in the pelvic area, especially if work on the fallopian tubes is involved. Microsurgery involves more than lenses; it involves principles of very gentle handling of tissue: keeping tissue moist, using small sutures, minimal operating time, and magnification as needed. Today, using microsurgical techniques, surgeons are able to achieve a better than 60 percent pregnancy rate with tubal reversals in sterilized women.

About the same time that microsurgery came to infertility, the surgical laser was developed for use in gynecology. In precision, the surgical laser exceeds all other forms of surgery. It allows the surgeon to reach inaccessible tissues, even reflecting beams around corners with mirrors. As it cuts, the laser damages only a few cells on either side of the impact site and it seals bleeding, thereby preventing new adhesion formation. Operating time is lessened and recovery time is faster. The CO_2 laser is now the most versatile one used in surgery. It can be tuned to penetrate or to merely prick a surface. Dr. Joseph Bellina of the Omega Institute in New Orleans was the first to use laser microsurgery on the female reproductive tract in 1974. His work with the laser on blocked fallopian tubes has been extremely successful.

The medical community at large has been slow to accept both microsurgery and especially laser surgery. Some specialists feel there is no evidence that the laser is any better than electrocautery. It involves expensive equipment that requires many hours of special training to use properly. It goes without saying that neither of these procedures belongs in the nonspecialist area. If you wish to find out locations of clinics and specialists using these new techniques, RESOLVE has an excellent referral service.

PROBLEMS OF THE UTERUS AND CERVIX

Structural or functional problems of the uterus or cervix constitute the least common category of female infertility. Diagnosis is usually readily made by pelvic exam and hysterosalpingogram.

Uterine Problems

The uterus is a firm, pear-shaped organ in the nonpregnant state and is rarely the cause of infertility. What problems do exist are either a result of developmental abnormalities or acquired problems such as scarring and adhesions or fibroid tumors.

The most common developmental abnormality of the uterus is a *bicornuate uterus* where the uterus is "heart-shaped" and separated to some degree inside by a septum. Sometimes the septum is complete and divides the uterus in half; more commonly it is partial. Rarely, women are born with two complete uteri, two cervices, and even two vaginas. Infertility in any of these cases correlates to the volume of the uterine cavity and whether the uterus can expand to contain a full-term pregnancy. If the problem is just a septum, this can be surgically removed using the hysteroscope and laser surgery or simple cutting. If the problem is a double uterus, the surgical correction is more involved and aimed at creating one uterus big enough to support a pregnancy. In some cases the double uterus does not require surgery to accommodate a pregnancy.

Women whose mothers took the hormone DES in their first and second trimesters have a tendency toward structural defects of the uterus. The so-called T-shaped uterus is seen on a hysterosalpingogram. Some of these women have infertility or repeated miscarriages, while others are still able to bear children.

Any infection of the endometrium of the uterus can cause scar tissue and adhesions to form. Sometimes scarring is so severe that the sides of the uterus are stuck together (*Asherman's syndrome*). This can be treated by surgery through the hysteroscope and laser or traditional surgery on the scar tissue. A small balloon is placed in the uterus while healing takes place to keep the walls apart. Hormones may be given to encourage the endometrium to grow back. Chronic infection of the endometrium is called *endometritis* and may respond to antibiotics, or to a dilation and curettage (D&C) to remove the lining. Polyps may also be removed by D&C.

Fibroid tumors are the most common of uterine problems. These benign tumors occur in one in four women after the age of thirty. Sometimes they cause no problem at all; sometimes they interfere with proper implantation of the embryo and cause early miscarriage. At times their location may create an obstruction into one or both of the fallopian tubes. The doctor can usually feel fibroids and discover their location in a pelvic exam. An ultrasound will give their exact size and location. Treatment is not called for unless the tumors are causing heavy bleeding or are interfering with pregnancy. Fibroids are the most common reason women have hysterectomies today, but this does not usually have to be the case if childbearing is desired. Myomectomy, surgical removal of the fibroids, can be performed with either traditional or new laser surgery techniques.

Cervical Problems

About 10 percent of infertility problems can be traced to a problem of the cervix. Usually these are problems related to the cervical mucus. Normally the glands in the cervix produce great quantities of mucus around ovulation time to provide a nourishing and slightly alkaline medium for the sperm. If the mucus turns acidic for any reason, or if it is scanty and thick or infected, sperm will die upon contact. Infections can be cultured and treated with antibiotics. Small doses of estrogen can sometimes improve cervical mucus. Small polyps may be present that obstruct or impede sperm passage. These can be removed.

Recently there has been much debate over the role of sperm antibodies in cervical mucus. For an unknown reason, some women produce antibodies to sperm. A postcoital test will reveal normal mucus but immobilized sperm. Checking to see if the woman has antibodies involves sophisticated serum assays. Some doctors have prescribed low or even high doses of steroids to women to reduce this response, but results have not been encouraging. The more traditional approach of having the woman avoid all contact with her husband's sperm for a number of months by using condoms during intercourse has been largely abandoned as ineffective. While the antibody level may fall, the couple can have unprotected relations to try to achieve a pregnancy only a short period of time before the antibody level rises again.

If a cervical mucus problem cannot be eradicated, husband insemination into the uterus may be tried to bypass the problem altogether. Since semen may carry bacteria that cervical mucus usually screens out, this procedure may introduce infection into the women. New "sperm washing" techniques are being used where the sperm are separated from the semen by centrifuge and are resuspended in a neutral, sterile medium. This is then inserted into the uterus via a small catheter.

Cryosurgery (freezing) or electrosurgery to remove growths in the cervical canal may affect mucus production by scarring the glands. Some doctors treat this problem with intrauterine insemination; others have prescribed glyceryl guaiacolate, the active ingredient in cough syrup, which may increase mucus secretions (as it does in the rest of the body). The best lesson learned from this problem is prevention of future cervical damage by limiting use of cryosurgery and electrosurgery.

The cervix may be rendered incompetent to support pregnancy by previous instrumentation, such as abortion at a young age. The cervical os simply dilates prematurely and the pregnancy will be lost, often between the twelfth to twentieth week. The only symptom is a *painless* spontaneous abortion. Such a condition is difficult to predict until it has happened once. The doctor should monitor future pregnancies closely and if the cervix begins to dilate, a purse-string suture can be placed around the cervix to hold it tight. In extreme cases the woman may also need bed rest.

6. Causes and Treatment of Male Infertility

> Be ye fruitful and multiply,
> and fill the earth and subdue it.
>
> GENESIS 1:27

Approximately 35 percent of all infertility problems are a direct result of a male problem. Another 20 percent are "combined-couple problems" and often result from a low or borderline sperm count on the part of the man, and a slight problem with the woman. The diagnostic tests used to determine the problem(s) in the infertile couple are discussed in chapter 4. It is important to emphasize once again that the man should enter the investigation as soon as the woman does, since he has an equal chance of having a problem. Since the investigation of the woman can be extensive compared to a man's relatively few tests, it makes sense to know the man is fertile before subjecting the woman to these procedures. Likewise, treatment of the male is relatively standard, and either will be successful rather quickly or not. This makes a good case for treatment of any male problem before proceeding with the female investigation.

PROBLEMS OF SPERM PRODUCTION OR MATURATION

Sperm production and maturation is dependent upon complete coordination between the hypothalamus and pituitary of the brain and the sperm and testosterone-producing cells of the testicles. A problem at any level will affect the end result. Before discussing these uncommon hormonal imbalances, let's look at the *varicocele*, which is not exactly a sperm-production problem, but does affect sperm production. Varicoceles occur in 30 to 40 percent of infertile men. Many professionals believe they are the leading cause of infertility in men. Others do not acknowledge their impact on infertility, simply because it is not yet completely known by what mechanism infertility results, and why it seems to act selectively in some men and not in others.

Varicocele

A varicocele is a bundle of dilated veins similar to varicose veins, occurring most frequently on the left spermatic vein due to slight anatomical differences in the veins draining the testicles. Exactly how it may lead to infertility remains a mystery. One theory believes the pooling of distended veins in the area overheats the sperm-production cells of the testicles, and excess heat has been known to kill sperm. On the other hand, heat can also speed up sperm production, causing cells to divide too quickly and resulting in immature and deformed sperm. Another theory is that toxins from the renal vein above, which serves to drain the kidney, somehow back up into the varicocele and have a chemical deterrent on sperm production. All of these arguments are plagued by the fact that 10 percent of all men have a varicocele and not all of them experience infertility. What is more, the size of the varicocele seems to make little difference; a small one can be as damaging as a huge one. When the varicocele is surgically tied off in an infertile man, sperm production often improves. However, varicocele as a cause of infertility and surgery to treat it remain controversial.

The decision to have surgery is usually made if a varicocele is present and the semen analysis shows a low sperm count accompanied by numerous immature forms known as *spermatids*. Either local or general anesthesia can be used. The surgeon (generally a urologist) makes an incision in the groin, locates the spermatic cord, and isolates the spermatic artery and vas deferens from the veins. The surgeon then ties off the main trunk of veins above the varicocele. New collateral circulation will open up to carry blood away from the testicle. The man usually remains in the hospital for the day or overnight and can return to normal activities comfortably within a week. A new balloon procedure has been developed that allows the surgeon to insert a tiny device into the vein by skin puncture and inflate it, blocking the vein. Another new technique involves the usual incision but utilizes microsurgery to tie off the main trunk and injection of the smaller veins with a sclerosing agent, which blocks them.

Whichever technique is used, the man must wait three months before a change is evident in the sperm in his ejaculate. Some improvement is generally seen at that time if the surgery was successful, but the maximum recovery occurs within about six months. Studies show that semen quality improves in about 80 percent of men having the varicocele surgery, but only about half of these go on to impregnate their wives. Not surprisingly, the most successful patients are those who had higher sperm counts (10 to 20 million per cc or more) before surgery. The overall success rate for this procedure makes it the most effective of all fertility treatments available to men.

Hormonal Problems

Sperm formation in the testicles is under endocrine control. The hypothalamus secretes a releasing hormone that acts on the pituitary, causing release of follicular stimulating hormone (FSH) and luteinizing hormone (LH). LH acts on the Leydig's cells in the testicles to produce testosterone. FSH acts upon the Sertoli cells to stimulate production of sperm cells. Presence of testosterone in the blood serum circulates the message back to the hypothalamus that enough LH is present. As sperm are produced, a substance called "inhibin" is released into the system and causes a decrease in FSH production. Drugs used to stimulate fertility by increasing sperm production can act at the hypothalamic-pituitary level or at the testicular level.

Clomiphene citrate is used in men in much the same fashion as it is used in women. The drug is an antiestrogen that blocks hypothalamic receptor sites. The hypothalamus does not react to rising serum testosterone by shutting off its releasing hormone and the pituitary is stimulated to go on producing more LH and FSH. LH increases stimulation of the Leydig's cells and increases the testosterone level. FSH also rises and stimulates more sperm production. Treatment with low doses of clomiphene extend over several months. Low doses are used since sperm production takes 74 days to be completed and prolonged therapy is needed. One common regimen is for the man to take 25 mg (½ tablet) for 25 nights, then stop 5 days and repeat. This dose keeps side effects to a minimum. Possible side effects are visual disturbances, liver damage, and scarring of the seminiferous tubules in the testicles. After two months the patient is checked to see if the LH and testosterone levels have risen. FSH, while it will rise, should remain within normal limits. If levels respond, the sperm count and motility are also expected to improve, but even without improvement, treatment may go on for up to a year. If the FSH level becomes abnormally high, without an improvement in the sperm production, a primary fault of the testicle is the problem and treatment is stopped. Success rates vary. One study showed improvement in 45 out of 57 men treated. The fertility rate for those who responded was 40 percent. Other studies are not as encouraging. Clomiphene seems to work best at improving motility.

Tamoxifin is a drug similar in action to clomiphene. When used at a dosage of 20 mg per day for six months, it causes a rise in the serum LH,

FSH, and testosterone levels. However there is less evidence that it is as effective as clomiphene in increasing sperm quality.

These treatments depend upon a normal hypothalamic-pituitary axis. If the patient does not have a normal hypothalamus, but has a normal pituitary, medical treatment involves giving LH and FSH directly, bypassing the brain level altogether. Human menopausal gonadotropin (HMG), sold under the brand name of Pergonal, was approved in 1981 for use in male as well as female infertility. The usual dose is 3 to 12 ampules injected weekly. For normal sperm production to be achieved (where possible) HCG has to be given by injection once a week as well. Once normal sperm production has been achieved, it can be maintained with HCG alone. Since the vast majority of infertile men have a normal hypothalamus, this treatment is uncommon. Some doctors have tried giving Pergonal or HCG to men with a normal hypothalamus, but since it involves twice-weekly, expensive injections, there is a strong case for using clomiphene, which is oral and equally effective.

If a male is found to have a high prolactin level, bromocriptine may be used to lower the level. High prolactin levels in either men or women have an adverse effect on fertility. Use of this drug in infertile men with normal prolactin levels appears to have a limited, experimental role.

Teslac is a synthetic male hormone that acts directly upon the testicle. The drug appears to interfere with the process by which testosterone is converted to estrogen. If this process is stopped within the testicle, it leads to sustained high intratesticular testosterone levels. These high levels may aid in development and maturation of the spermatocytes.

Other Problems

There are a variety of problems that can result in damage to the sperm-producing cells of the testicles. Mumps in the male after the age of puberty can lead to *mumps orchitis*, which is a disease that can destroy the sperm-producing cells. In 70 percent of these cases, only one testicle is affected, but some men are left permanently sterile from this disease. If no sperm are present on semen analysis, there is no treatment. If some sperm-producing cells remain functional, treatment with clomiphene may be tried. Sexually transmitted diseases rarely get past the urethra of the male, but in about 2 percent of the cases infection will get as far as the epididymis. Treatment consists of either penicillin or tetracycline, depending on the organism.

Trauma to the testicles is fortunately rare, but it can result from occurrences such as sports injuries or accidents. Ruptured vessels reduce the oxygen supply to the sperm-producing cells and may cause them to die. Such injuries require immediate surgical attention. Prevention by use of sports protective cups or supporters is advised in all strenuous sports. *Torsion* is a rare, spontaneous event where a testicle twists on its own blood supply. This is very painful and sudden and requires immediate attention. If the testicle is not released within six hours, it will die. The testicles are like the eyes, in that one will often have a "sympathetic" response to injury of the other. Therefore, damage to one testicle may result in complete sterility. Surgical injury can threaten the blood supply to one or both testicles. Hernia repair or surgery to correct undescended testicles both come very close to the spermatic cord, which carries the blood supply to the testicles. Permanent death to the testicle can result if the blood supply is inadvertently cut off.

There are a few problems of sperm production that a man is simply born with. *Sertoli cell–only syndrome* is a rare condition where the sperm-producing cells are missing. This seems to be a congenital problem and one for which there is no treatment. *Klinefelter's syndrome* is a congenital disorder of the sex chromosomes in which the man will have at least one extra X chromosome in his XY complement. It is analogous to Turner's syndrome of the woman, in that the person is genetically sterile but appears normal in every other way. Some men with this problem have small testicles and slightly enlarged breasts. A testosterone supplement can be given to supply the missing male hormone, but there is no other treatment. Undescended testicles (cryptorchidism) occurs in about 1 in 200 male babies. One or both testicles remain within the body and do not descend into the scrotal sac as they should. This diagnosis can be made at birth and is usually treated by eighteen months of age if the testicles do not descend on their own. HCG is given first to see if the testicles will descend; surgery is done if they don't, usually by the age of two. If the child reaches puberty without treatment, permanent damage can be done to the sperm-producing cells. Sons of mothers who took DES while pregnant have an increased incidence of abnormal semen analysis. This is an area still being researched. Finally, many environmental factors may affect sperm production, either temporarily or permanently. Stress, excessive heat, chemical toxins, drugs (certain antihypertensive and antidepressives, certain ulcer medications, marijuana, alcohol), diet, radiation, and altitude have all been shown to have an effect on sperm production. The man is far more at risk than the woman is to environmental factors because he is constantly producing his sperm cells. But the man also has the advantage of "recovery" after most of these factors are removed, unless sperm-producing cells have been permanently injured. Indeed, semen analysis might be seen one day as an important industrial monitoring test (exposure to hazards) and as a general indicator of health and well-being.

PROBLEMS OF SPERM MOTILITY

Motility is thought by many to be the most important factor in the semen analysis. Even a very nominal count may be fertile if the sperm are vigorously motile.

Drugs that attempt to improve sperm motility are some of the same already mentioned. Clomiphene will increase motility in about 50 percent of cases. HCG, at a dose of 2,500 units intramuscular (IM) every 5 days for four months increased motility for 16 out of 17 patients in one study. When motility is impaired because semen is too thick, small amounts of estrogen and vitamin C have also been used to reduce viscosity.

Semen-volume problems often fall into this category. Too little semen may result in high viscosity of the ejaculate. Too much volume may dilute the sperm cells and many may be lost from the vagina. In the first case, sperm cells may be separated from the semen in a specimen by centrifuging and then added to a neutral medium that serves as the semen vehicle. This can then be placed into the cervical area by artificial insemination (husband), also called AIH. In the case of a fertile man with a high volume of semen, the ejaculate is collected in two containers—ideally the first few waves in the first and the remainder in the second. Since the vast majority of motile sperm are found in the first waves of ejaculate, and the latter part is mostly semen, an ejaculate which is of smaller volume can be gathered. This is also placed into the woman via a catheter in artificial insemination by the husband.

Prostate infections can also pose fertility problems. The man's sperm count and motility will be depressed while the infection is rampant, but they return to normal when treatment is effective. The prostate is very hard to treat. Even after antibiotic therapy, bacteria can remain in the multiple lobes of the prostate and cause recurrent flare-ups. Any illness of the male accompanied by high fever may temporarily result in low sperm production. Usually, if the testicles were not directly involved in the infection, sperm production will rebound within three months.

The problem of the woman's antibodies against the man's sperm has already been discussed, but apparently a man may also create antibodies against his own sperm. The sperm may be "good," but they are clumped together so they can't swim. To remedy this, a variation of the "sperm washing" technique is employed, wherein the sperm are centrifuged to separate them from semen and are resuspended in fresh media three times in an effort to wash off all the antibodies. Finally they are collected, suspended in a fresh medium, and inseminated into the woman.

PROBLEMS OF BLOCKAGE OF THE SPERM TRANSPORT SYSTEM

Absence of Vasa Deferentia

In less than 5 percent of infertile men there is congenital absence of the vasa deferentia, which carry the sperm from the testicles to the area from where they are ejaculated. There is no way to re-create the vas surgically if it does not exist. Some efforts have been made to create a small pouch between the epididymis and the vas to collect sperm, which might then be withdrawn by a needle and artificially inseminated into the woman. To date no pregnancies have resulted from this highly experimental technique. Absence of the vas would be revealed by vasography after a semen analysis showed no sperm cells.

Vasectomy

It may seem odd to include vasectomy, which is a voluntary sterilization procedure chosen by many men, in this section. Each year, despite being counseled that this surgery should be thought of as "permanent," men opt to reverse vasectomies. A large number are men who have divorced their original partners and remarried younger women who want to have children. Reversing vasectomy, called *vasovasotomy*, in the hands of a skilled micro-surgeon, is quite successful. The success will depend on the amount of damage done to the vas where it was tied off and seems also to be affected by the length of time the man has been sterilized. Success rates for vas reconstruction, as seen by viable sperm in the ejaculate, vary from 60 to 80 percent. As usual, pregnancy rates are not as high, ranging from 30 to 35 percent. It is suspected that the difference between presence of sperm and successful pregnancy rate is due to the development of antibodies. Men who are considering vasectomy as a form of birth control should always be counseled carefully and told that it may be irreversible.

Blockage of the Epididymis

Most blockages in the epididymis are the result of an infection or a congenital defect. If the blockage is located near where the epididymis enters the vas, it is easier to repair. The tubules of the epididymis are very thin and tightly coiled, making it virtually impossible to unravel the structure, locate, and mend a blockage. If the blockage is near the vas, microsurgery may give about a 20 percent chance of success. Chances are minimal if the blockage is elsewhere.

Blockage of the Ejaculatory Ducts

Infection may cause blockage in the ejaculatory ducts. The culprit is usually gonorrhea. The surgeon must work through the urethra with a cystoscope because these channels are buried deep in the prostate gland. The scope locates the blockage and attempts to dilate it with a narrow tube.

PROBLEMS OF DEPOSITION OF SPERM

Problems of sexual technique are really a problem of the couple, not just the man. But, nature has contrived that it is the man, not the woman, who must obtain and maintain an erection and achieve an ejaculation within the vagina in order for sperm to fertilize her egg. The woman's role in sex is really quite passive if she wishes it to be. She does not have to become aroused (although lack of lubrication may cause discomfort or pain during intercourse) and she does not have to achieve orgasm to get pregnant. One would hope, in a loving couple, that she is as involved as her partner, but one can readily see that much of the burden, in sexual technique, is upon the male.

Timing and Frequency of Sex

We will begin with an obvious statement: In order to achieve pregnancy a couple must be having intervaginal sex. Every now and then a doctor sees a couple who have actually never achieved consummation. They may, through lack of education, physical deformities, or obesity, be practicing interlabial sex. Education will often solve the problem very quickly. Sometimes the problem is as simple as improper timing of relations around the fertile period. Most doctors have seen classic cases of couples who "save up sperm" all month until the rise in the temperature chart is seen and then they jump into bed. They are, in effect, practicing birth control, since the rise in the chart comes 1 to 2 days after ovulation and the ovum may live as little as 12 hours. Sometimes incompatibility of job schedules or frequent travel makes it difficult for couples to get together around the fertile time of the month. Most doctors gently suggest that the couple try to have relations every other day around the time of ovulation. If ovulation is expected on day 14, for example, relations on days 11, 13, and 15 would give excellent coverage, since sperm may live up to 48 hours. Too frequent sex is occasionally a problem. This may actually result in a lowered sperm count. Very infrequent relations may also have a bad effect on sperm count and motility, as sperm in storage in the system tend to die. The important thing in educating couples about timing and frequency is to state that their sexual practices may be whatever they wish throughout the month, but that sex every other day at ovulation time gives the best chance for pregnancy.

A practice of Orthodox Judaism sometimes creates a catch-22 on timing relations for ovulation. The woman may not have intercourse while she is menstruating (this may be up to 7 days) and for 7 bloodless days following the menstrual period. At the end of this time the woman immerses herself in a ritual bath (*mikvah*), after which intercourse is permitted. In some couples, the period of abstinence coincides with the fertile time. To change this practice, rabbinic permission must be sought.

Impotence

If the problem is one of impotence, the inability of the man to maintain an erection, careful history taking must try to reveal if the problem is a transient one, related to stress or emotional problems, or if it is one of longer duration, which may be due to underlying medical problems, use of certain drugs or alcohol, or deep-seated psychological factors. Many doctors and therapists are guilty of ascribing all impotence to psychological factors, therefore overlooking physical causes. Diabetes is a disease that frequently leads to impotence in the adult male. As many as half of all diabetic men will experience this problem. Certain antihypertensive medications can lead to impotence. Should this be a side effect, the man should ask about possible alternative medications, since there are many to choose from and some do not have this unfortunate side effect. The use of narcotics, certain tranquilizers in the phenothiazine class, drugs in the monamine oxidase-inhibitor family (MOA), and alcohol can all lead to impotence or loss of libido.

A variation on this problem is retrograde ejaculation, where potency is achieved, but the man cannot ejaculate from the penis. Instead the semen is forced backward into the bladder. This problem is usually neurological and may be caused by diabetes or the drugs mentioned above as well. If changes in drug therapy cannot solve the problem, attempts can be made at artificial insemination. First the man must void and the bladder is rinsed via a catheter with a solution to neutralize it and make it hospitable to sperm. The man then masturbates to orgasm and the sperm are voided into a collection jar, washed, resuspended in neutral medium, and inseminated into the woman.

Premature Ejaculation

Occasionally a man will be unable to control his orgasm, to the point where any stimulation of the penis will cause a hair-trigger reaction. He may be unable to deposit semen within the woman because he simply cannot wait long enough for penetration. This is not only an infertility problem, but a problem of sexual satisfaction, since the woman is almost never able to achieve her own arousal and orgasm as quickly. The work of Masters and Johnson in *Human Sexual Response*, published in 1966, was a landmark work of explicit sexual functioning and malfunctioning and some therapeutic methods to overcome problems. Their exercises, by which a man can learn to control his orgasm, have proved extremely helpful in overcoming this problem and leading both to fertility (for those who wish it) and increased mutual sexual satisfaction.

Coital Technique

It cannot be overstated that the couple may do what they please in the way of sexual pleasuring at any time of the month. If they are really eager to enhance fertility, then they need worry only about the midpoint of the woman's cycle, when certain practices may lead to a better chance of pregnancy. First, the optimal position for placing sperm at the neck of the cervix is the woman on her back and the man on top. Some doctors recommend a pillow under the woman's hips to increase the angle and keep more sperm inside. No artificial lubricants should be used, since almost all (Vaseline, K-Y jelly, mineral oil) have a spermicidal effect. If the woman does not lubricate well with foreplay, saliva is readily available and not harmful to sperm. Some others recommend raw egg white as a safe lubricant. Precoital douches that scent or flavor the vagina are possibly harmful to sperm and should be avoided. After the man has ejaculated, the woman should draw her knees up and remain on her back for 15 to 20 minutes to give the sperm the maximum chance to pass through the cervical opening and swim upward toward the tubes, where fertilization takes place. After this, she may urinate and bathe if she wishes, but she should never douche.

Ideally, timing of sexual relations to achieve pregnancy should be every other day around the time of ovulation (as demonstrated by previous cycles of basal body temperature [BBT] charts, or the new urine-testing kits that predict ovulation). Once the rise is seen in the temperature chart, ovulation has occurred and sexual practice may return to the frequency, position, and imagination of the couple. Since there is a great deal of pressure to "perform" at midcycle for both partners, sometimes alternatives to intercourse such as massage, cuddling, and nonsexual embracing are a welcome change of pace.

Some women (especially those with endometriosis or previous pelvic infections) may experience pain during intercourse, called *dyspareunia*, and this may cause them to tense up as the man enters. This spasm of vaginal muscles is called *vaginismus* and may be so strong that it prevents penetration by the man, or makes it very painful for both of them. An alternate position, which is more comfortable for such women, is the rear-entry position. If the woman kneels and places her face and shoulders down upon the pillow, entry is often painless and sperm are still delivered to the cervical area and will remain there as long as she lies in this position. Frigidity, or inability of the woman to achieve orgasm, is not a known cause of infertility. However, couples experiencing this problem may wish to read or consult experts to help in increasing their mutual sexual satisfaction. The goal of any doctor or therapist who gives sexual education and counseling should be the improvement of the couple's mutual sexual satisfaction and personal communication, not just enhanced fertility.

7. Pregnancy Loss

What we have done will not be lost to all eternity.
Everything ripens at its own time and becomes
fruit at its hour.

DIVYAVADANA

Of all the tragedies of infertility, miscarriage and stillbirth stand apart as among the most acutely painful of experiences. Sometimes a couple have struggled years to achieve the goal of pregnancy, only to be robbed of the real goal—a liveborn child.

UNDERSTANDING MISCARRIAGE

The term *miscarriage* will be used in this book instead of the medical term *abortion* to eliminate possible confusion between induced or therapeutic abortion and spontaneous loss of pregnancy. About 1 in every 6 pregnancies ends in miscarriage, a fact not commonly known. Studies quote rates as low as 10 percent and as high as 40 percent, so there is clearly no consensus on the miscarriage rate, just as with so many areas of infertility. One study claims that as many as 70 percent of all conceptions fail to achieve viability, and of these, 50 percent are lost prior to the first missed menstrual period, when a woman may not even know she is pregnant. However, of those miscarriages that occur, about 75 percent occur in the first trimester of pregnancy (weeks 1 through 12) and these are frequently unavoidable. In the remaining 25 percent of cases, miscarriage takes place in the second trimester of pregnancy (weeks 12 to 24), when causes are more complex and possibly preventable. Any fetus that survives into the third trimester has passed the arbitrary "age of viability" (set at 24 to 26 weeks of gestation) and is termed a premature birth if born alive or a stillbirth if born dead. Premature babies have a statistical chance of survival that improves dramatically with every week of gestation after the age of viability.

Miscarriage can be divided into the following categories:

Threatened miscarriage. If a woman has vaginal bleeding or spotting in pregnancy, which may or may not be accompanied by minor cramps, she is seen as threatening to miscarry. The cervix is still closed and the process may stop by itself or very rarely by medical intervention. It usually, however, progresses to the next category.

Inevitable miscarriage. If the process has gone so far that termination of the pregnancy cannot be prevented, it is termed inevitable. Bleeding will be more profuse and usually brighter red in color and cramps more intense, equaling labor contractions and dilating the cervix. The products of conception may be expelled completely, or they may be incomplete.

Incomplete miscarriage. When only part of the products of conception has been passed and some tissue is retained, the miscarriage is incomplete. Bleeding will continue and may be profuse until the remaining tissue is removed. The doctor will generally do a dilation and curettage (D&C) at this time.

Complete miscarriage. Complete expulsion of the products of conception is called complete miscarriage. Some doctors do a D&C in either case as a safeguard against any possible retained tissue and subsequent risk of bleeding or infection.

Missed miscarriage. In a missed miscarriage the fetus dies in the uterus but is not expelled. The term is generally applied to those cases where two or more months have elapsed between fetal death and expulsion. The symptoms are amenorrhea (absence of periods), cessation of the signs of "feeling pregnant," and failure of the uterus to expand as it would in normal pregnancy. The treatment is either D&C or induction of labor, depending on the gestation of the fetus.

Habitual miscarriage. When a woman has a history of three or more successive miscarriages, it is termed habitual miscarriage.

THE COURSE OF A MISCARRIAGE

One of the reasons a miscarriage is so frightening is that the couple are rarely prepared for it and often do not understand the physiological events that are happening. This is, of course, compounded by all the feelings that accompany the loss of a pregnancy. Here is the usual sequence of events:

The woman begins to spot or bleed vaginally. The bleeding is often brownish in color. She may continue to spot or bleed on and off for several days or even for several weeks. Because bleeding in the first trimester of pregnancy is fairly common (although never normal), the doctor may not be particularly alarmed when the woman first calls. In many cases the pregnancy continues safely and bleeding stops. In the case of any person who is "at risk" (see pages 74 to 75) the doctor may want to see her or advise bed rest and a period of watchful waiting. Bleeding in the second trimester is much more actively monitored.

If the miscarriage is going to progress, the next sign is usually increased bleeding of a brighter red color. Uterine cramps may begin. The woman should call her doctor if either of these signs occurs and should be hospitalized if possible. Bleeding may become profuse, with large clots and a frightening volume of blood. Cramps may increase to the intensity of labor contractions.

Finally, tissue will be passed, either partially or completely, that is obviously not a clot and may be distinguishable as products of conception. This should be saved in a container for pathology to examine as it may give some clue as to the cause of miscarriage. In very early miscarriage, this tissue may be lost within a blood clot because it is very small.

After the uterine contents are expelled, the uterus tries to clamp down and bleeding should subside. Some doctors advise a D&C anyway to be sure all tissue is out and to reduce the risk of infection or hemorrhage. One possible complication of doing a D&C is Asherman's syndrome (see page 57). The D&C is performed with the woman under short-term or local anesthesia. Physical recovery is usually swift and the patient may go home the same day. Bleeding similar to normal menstrual flow will occur for about one week. The breasts may be very tender and may even lactate a little. A firm brassiere will offer support and discourages milk production. The doctor will usually want to examine the woman in one month's time, after which normal sexual relations can resume (if not earlier). The doctor will also give advice on when the next pregnancy may be attempted and what was the possible cause of the previous pregnancy ending in miscarriage.

This sequence describes merely the physical events of miscarriage. The emotional turmoil and pain may be intense, as the following quote attests:

> We did not understand what was happening and why, why it was happening to us. Did this mean there was something wrong with one of us? Did this mean we could never have children? Had I done something wrong in the early months to cause this miscarriage? We were so frightened by the amount and the look of what was pouring out of me. . . . It wasn't bad enough we were losing our baby, but in the midst of all that pain, we had to stay strong enough to deal with all that blood.

THE CAUSES OF MISCARRIAGE

Much is still unknown about the causes (and therefore the treatment) of miscarriage. On one point there seems to be agreement: Miscarriage is rarely the result of an emotional shock, a fall, or other environmental factors (with chemicals and toxins excepted and discussed later). In a healthy pregnancy, the fetus in utero is in a veritable fortress. Afloat in a sea of fluid, wrapped securely in a membranous sac, and surrounded by a firm muscular mass and beyond that, soft visceral organs, the fetus has been known to survive falls of mothers out second-story windows, serious car accidents, strokes, and all manner of emotional stresses. The reason to emphasize what *doesn't* cause a miscarriage is that a couple usually review their lives in an attempt to create a cause-and-effect relationship for the loss of a baby. There are reasons why miscarriages happen, but most are outside of environmental control.

Genetic Error

Almost 50 percent of first-trimester miscarriages are the result of an embryo that has not developed properly. Sometimes called a "blighted pregnancy," such a mass of cells will continue to divide and will implant and grow for a time but does not have the ability to survive longer than about 12 weeks. There is no treatment for this random event in nature except to expel the conceptus and try again. This fact is behind the sometimes "heartless" attitude of the doctor who refuses to intervene with medications or even bed rest, but rather encourages activity to bring on the miscarriage if it is inevitable. Such an event is unlikely to occur again in the lifetime of a couple, but if they are at risk for genetic disorders, or if they suffer repeated losses of this type, further genetic studies should be done on each partner to determine their situation. Genetic studies can also be done on the D&C material.

Hormonal Problems

Abnormal hormone levels in the woman may lead to early miscarriage if the lining of the uterus is improperly prepared for implantation and development of the conceptus. Luteal phase defects (described in chapter 5) are one type of hormonal problem that can be readily identified and treated. Progesterone support may be given in the form of vaginal suppositories or injections to get the pregnancy safely along to the stage where the placenta takes over progesterone production. Some doctors feel this has not been proven to work and advise against women taking any hormones during pregnancy. Other hormone problems may come from thyroid or adrenal gland imbalance. Women with diabetes are also at risk of miscarriage from hormone imbalance.

One problem with hormonal problems is that they may not show up until the miscarriage is threatening, and at that point it is hard to tell if the imbalance is cause or effect of the problem. For example, to give progesterone to a woman who is already bleeding may just prolong the miscarriage of an already dead fetus. Hormonal imbalances are best diagnosed in the nonpregnant state so the pregnancy can be monitored as "high risk" from its beginning.

Structural Problems of the Uterus

Miscarriages due to structural problems generally take place in the second trimester of pregnancy. Structural problems of the uterus usually cause miscarriage by interfering with the growth of the fertilized egg. Uterine fibroids (myomas) are noncancerous growths in the muscular layer of the uterus which can actually block the fallopian tube(s) or impinge on implantation or fetal growth and cause miscarriage. If the woman has an unusual-shaped uterus, a heart-shaped, bicornuate, or the T-shaped uterus sometimes associated with DES exposure, implantation or fetal growth may be impaired. Asherman's syndrome, characterized by scar tissue inside the uterus, may be the result of poorly performed abortion, D&C, or infection of the endometrium. All of these structural problems can be readily diagnosed with hysterosalpingogram and/or hysteroscopy, and many are surgically correctable. Some women with mild forms of these disorders have successful pregnancies without treatment.

Structural Problems of the Cervix

A common cause of second-trimester or even third-trimester pregnancy is a weakened or *incompetent* cervix. This condition is usually acquired, not congenital, although it is sometimes seen with DES-exposed women. It may be the result of a previous pregnancy and a cervical tear left unrepaired, or be the result of too many dilations of the cervix for tests, therapeutic abortions, or previous miscarriages. The result is a cervix that does not remain firmly closed and weakens with the growing weight of the fetus. It dilates prematurely, allowing the membranes to rupture and the fetus to be lost. Fortunately, this problem can be successfully treated if diagnosed in time. A ring of sutures is stitched around the cervix in a "purse-string" procedure known as the *Shirodkar procedure* in honor of the Indian gynecologist who developed it. When true labor begins, the stitches are cut and dilation of the cervix proceeds normally.

Infections

Infections such as German measles (rubella), herpes simplex, and T-mycoplasma can affect fetal development and result in miscarriage. The diseases toxoplasmosis and listeriosis are also being studied for their role in miscarriage. Toxoplasmosis is particularly important to know about if the couple has a cat, because the organism is passed through cat feces. A woman who is pregnant should avoid cleaning a cat litter box. Women who are not immune to German measles should consider being vaccinated before pregnancy. It is advisable to wait three months after such immunization before attempting pregnancy. Women who have cultured positive for urea-plasma, T-mycoplasma, or chlamydia should receive treatment with the appropriate antibiotic before attempting pregnancy. The role of the herpes simplex virus is still being studied and may be a significant cause of previously unexplained miscarriages. It appears that it occurs even in women with no known history of herpes simplex infection.

Immunologic Causes

There is new research being done on the possibility that early miscarriage may result from an immunologic cause. Some women may respond to the developing fetus as a foreign protein and produce a substance that rejects the fetus, resulting in miscarriage. This theory remains to be proven, but research is progressing. It is also conjectured that some women fail to produce a substance that prevents rejection of the fetus.

Environmental Factors

Toxins in the workplace or home can lead to fetal damage or miscarriage. Chemicals such as solvents, insecticides, lead products, benzene, and mercury all seem to increase risk of miscarriage. Women who work around anesthesia while pregnant have a higher incidence of miscarriage. Studies have proved that excessive use of alcohol, cigarette smoking, marijuana, and caffeine can all affect fetal development and possibly result in miscarriage. Doctors recommend abstinence or extreme moderation of all these sub-stances. Use of any prescription or nonprescription drug during pregnancy should be cleared with the doctor. Some drugs are known to cross the placental barrier and get into the fetal system, while others are safe to take if necessary.

HIGH-RISK CANDIDATES FOR MISCARRIAGE

Couples who do not conceive readily seem to have a higher percentage of miscarriages than does the general population—some studies suggest as high as 40 percent. Therefore, any woman who is pregnant after a long siege of infertility should be managed by the doctor as a high-risk case, as she is carrying a very precious pregnancy. The infertility specialist usually keeps a close eye on such a patient until it has been confirmed that the pregnancy is in the uterus (not ectopic), that a heartbeat has been established (usually around the sixteenth week), and that all other signs indicate that the woman and fetus are in good health. At that point, the specialist who does not maintain an obstetrical practice will refer the woman to an obstetrician. Other women who should be considered high risk in pregnancy are those with diabetes, heart disease, high blood pressure, or a previous history of miscarriage or stillbirth.

THE EMOTIONAL IMPACT OF MISCARRIAGE

Beyond the pain of losing a longed-for baby, a miscarriage is a terrifying event to most couples for other reasons. It is usually completely unexpected. It may be over in a matter of minutes (in early pregnancy) or it may drag on for days or even weeks. A woman who first experiences spotting in pregnancy is usually told by her doctor that, while it is never "normal," it is relatively common and often the bleeding abates and a healthy pregnancy continues. The couple experience alternate states of hoping and despair as they wait to see which outcome will be their fate.

> I found a medical book on obstetrics that had several pages on all the freaky things that can happen—like a woman menstruating every month for nine months and still a healthy baby pops out. I was particularly reassured by a little phrase "implantation bleeding," which the book said could occur in the first few months and was just the baby nestling deeper in his uterine fortress. When my bleeding changed from spotting to flow, and then to bright red flow, I still clung to this absurd thought of implantation bleeding. I remember bargaining with God over some point of virtue which I promised I would change if only He would let us have this baby. My husband was home with me, but we wandered in such separate, tense circles that we scarcely communicated. When the cramping began in earnest, we headed for the hospital. Even then I kept thinking, "This can't happen to us. We deserve a baby so much. God won't let this happen." I aborted an hour later—a 13-week fetus.

For both the man and the woman, the sight of blood, especially if it is thick with clots, may be unnerving. Both are often surprised by the intensity of the "cramps" experiences as the cervix thins and dilates. The woman is actually in labor, and depending on the gestation, it may take a number of hours of strong contractions to dilate the cervix fully enough to expel the fetus. The welfare of the fetus in first- or second-trimester miscarriage is usually not in question, as it has not reached the age of viability outside the uterus and has no chance to survive. The woman will be medicated to ease her pain and calm her down. In last-trimester deliveries, medication is often withheld in order not to depress the respirations of the premature infant if it should be born alive. This makes a premature birth more traumatic to the already upset patient.

> There was a special agony in miscarrying late in pregnancy (seven months). It was the loss of someone known, felt, anticipated, yet curiously unseen—whose kicks and thrusts had delighted us for several months. Physically, my wife's body was prepared to nurse a baby. Her breasts swelled with milk and ached for days. We both wondered silently by what sense of justice such a misfortune befell us—what social, religious, or biological rules we had violated. . . .

In the crisis of a miscarriage or stillbirth and the subsequent grieving, the man is often a forgotten or neglected person. True, he was not pregnant in his body, but the lost child and the dreams that accompanied it were very much of his making. Most attention is turned to the woman, and the man is expected to be strong, supportive, and reassuring.

> I went to work the day after the miscarriage, not because I felt like it but because I seemed to be in the way at the hospital and it was too lonely at home. At lunch a secretary stopped and said she had heard about it. "Give my condolences to your wife," she said (and what about *me?*). Later a guy took me out for a few beers to cheer me up. "A stud like you will have her pregnant again in no time" (and what about *this* time?).

A miscarriage today rarely poses a threat to the life of a woman, but many couples admit to having feared the woman's life would be lost. Literature and soap operas are filled with deathbed scenes following miscarriage and stillbirth. Another common fear is that hysterectomy will have to be performed. This is never done unless hemorrhage persists in the face of all heroics of the medical team. One other fear often expressed is that "this means we can never have children." A miscarriage or stillbirth is not a prediction for the future; it is the loss of the current pregnancy. Time and medical advice will indicate whether there is any reason to be concerned for the future.

HOW HOSPITALS COULD HELP

Complicating the physical and emotional events of a miscarriage is the fact that the woman is usually hospitalized. The imposition of hospital rules and unfamiliar personnel robs the event of privacy and may inhibit natural feelings. Hospitals vary in their protocol for miscarrying patients. Many consider them obstetrical admissions and therefore send them to the labor area to miscarry and to the postpartum floor for recovery. Hospital administrators justify this policy by pointing out that the obstetrical area is considered "clean," whereas the gynecology area often deals with infections and cancer and is considered less clean. The patient who is miscarrying is not generally infected and it is in her best interest to be admitted to the cleanest possible area. However, this placement takes no account of the emotional impact on the woman who must be in close proximity to laboring and newly delivered mothers.

> Seeing a bassinet in the delivery room as I was being "prepped" for a D&C really blew my mind. I started screaming, "Get that thing out of here—*there is no baby!*" At that point they sedated me. When I woke up I was in a recovery room next to a newly delivered woman. She asked me, "Did you have a boy or a girl?"

If the woman must be admitted to the obstetrical area of the hospital, then some considerations are in order. At the very least, the couple who have just lost a baby should be screened from laboring or newly delivered patients. They should have a room of their own, as far as possible from the nursery area. Some sort of special indicator, known to all staff, should be posted on the door or bed to alert the multitudes who drift through a hospital room in the course of their work (housekeeping, nutritionists, aides, students) that this is a couple who have lost a baby. Unfortunately, this sort of tagging may lead to its own problems, as everyone from the person who washes the floors to the volunteer delivering flowers may feel compelled to remark on the loss and offer platitudes such as, "It's probably a blessing—the baby wouldn't have been normal," "I know someone who had *eight* miscarriages before she bore a child," and the ever popular, "You'll be pregnant again before you know it." The couple should be assigned to the minimum number of caretakers, with as much continuity as possible during their stay. In family-centered maternity care, the husband should be considered a part of the admission, not merely a "visitor" and allowed 24-hour access to his wife. Other visitors should be restricted to those the couple feel capable of receiving.

THE NEED TO GRIEVE

A couple who have lost a baby, at whatever stage of gestation, need to grieve. Grief means crying, and crying is not easy for many hospital staff to witness, as they often equate this normal and necessary emotion with "suffering." It is unfortunate that doctors and nurses often request sedation or tranquilizing medications which dull the senses and blunt the grief process, so they do not have to deal with it during the hospitalization. This delay may cause the couple to abort the grief process in the place they are really safest to experience it, for a sympathetic nurse or counselor is often available to them in a medical center, but not at home. Since grief is a frightening feeling to many people, once they return home they may simply try to go on as if nothing had happened. In early miscarriage there is no body to bury, no social ritual to deal with the loss, and the couple have a sense that the experience was "unreal."

Grief cleanses the wound of loss so that it may heal. In order to gain control of their lives and recover, the couple first need to *lose* control and experience their feelings. Everyone, from family and friends to hospital staff, seems to work at cross-purposes to this. Privacy is often denied. Reminders of children at home or assurances of future pregnancies are offered as "comfort." What needs to be understood by all is that *the death of this particular child is being experienced.*

> I could not cry when I lost the baby. I was in a strange bed with an intravenous in my arm and a real "high" from the morphine they had given me. It was just like a surrealistic nightmare. My husband was not with me. He had been sent home at eight just like all the visitors. I wished so much he could have stayed and held me. When I woke in the morning I was terribly depressed, but still I could not cry. I had decided to keep my grief for home. I had a D&C that morning. When I was in the recovery area, coming out of my anesthetic, I heard a woman crying as if her heart would break. In my fog I kept wondering why no one was helping her. Then I realized it was me.

The man is half of the grieving couple, but he is often forgotten, banned from access to his wife, and expected to be the stalwart pillar around which new hopes for the future must somehow rally. Out of this comes a double sadness: The man may stifle all his longings to grieve; the woman may never know how deeply he felt.

> What did I *want* to do? Hell, I wanted to get in the bed with her and hold her close and cry like a baby! What did I *do?* I watched her cry from across the room—so many people coming in and out . . . then I said the hell with it and left and got roaring drunk. I don't think she will ever forgive me for that.

The classic Robert Frost poem *"Home Burial"* tells the story of differing grieving styles. The story is of a woman who loses her firstborn child and locks her husband out of her grief, feeling he could not understand. In confrontation she hurls these words:

> If you had any feelings, you that dug
> With your own hand—how could you—his little grave;
> I saw you from that very window there,
> Making the gravel leap and leap in air,
> Leap up, like that, and land so lightly
> And roll back down the mound beside the hole.
> I thought, who is this man? I didn't know you.
> And I crept down the stairs and up the stairs
> To look again and still your spade kept lifting.
> Then you came in. I heard your rumbling voice
> Out in the kitchen, and I don't know why,
> But I went near to see with my own eyes.
> You could sit there with the stains on your shoes
> Of the fresh earth from your own baby's grave
> And talk about your everyday concerns. . . .
>
> I can repeat the very words you were saying.
> "Three foggy mornings and one rainy day
> Will rot the best birch fence a man can build."
> Think of it, talk like that at such a time!*

The elements that facilitate a couple's grief are these: unlimited access to each other, privacy from all but essential care tenders and visitors, a nurturing environment, reflective discussion and listening by others, and warm physical contact.

> The only thing that anyone said to me that felt any good was this: An old nurse said, "That's right, you cry. There is nothing anyone can say just now that will make you feel better." And she sat with me silently for a long time, her big, warm hand on my shoulder.

STILLBIRTH

Stillbirth is a very unusual event in these days of good prenatal care and closely monitored labor and delivery. It is predictably higher where these benefits are not available to patients.

---

* From "Home Burial" in *The Poetry of Robert Frost*, Edward Connery Lathem, ed. Reprinted by permission of Holt, Rhinehart & Winston, Publishers.

A stillbirth is usually the result of loss of the fetus's oxygen supply in the uterus. This can be the result of severe compression of the umbilical cord during labor, premature separation of the placenta (a maternal crisis as well, as there is profuse bleeding), or separation of the umbilical cord from the placenta. There are also congenital abnormalities of the heart and/or lungs which make oxygenation of the baby impossible once the placental supply is lost. Babies this happens to succumb immediately upon birth when the cord is cut.

The management of a stillbirth must vary with the situation. If the baby is known to be dead before delivery, anesthesia and delivery by the least hazardous route to the woman is advisable. If the baby gets into distress during labor, an immediate C section will be ordered. The husband should be in attendance if possible. The baby, once delivered, should be handled in a reverent and careful manner. The couple are facilitated in their grief if they can see and hold their dead baby for a while. When autopsy is planned to discover the cause of death, this should be done *after* the couple have had a chance to say their good-byes. Since the woman is invariably delivered in an obstetrical unit and is sent to the postpartum floor to recover, it is helpful if she can be isolated from those having normal labor and if she can have a private room away from the nursery afterward. All the considerations mentioned in the miscarriage discussion apply even more so in stillbirth, since the recovery phase will be longer.

Following a stillbirth, the woman is in a postpartum condition. She may have an episiotomy if the birth was vaginal or abdominal incision and sutures if the birth was cesarean. She will be physically exhausted if she labored long and will have lochia, the flow of afterbirth, for a week or so. Her breasts will swell with milk on the second or third day after delivery and will be painfully taut for several days, as there is no baby to nurse. (In many other countries there is the age-old profession of wet-nursing, in which a woman who has lost her baby hires out to nurture another child in need of breast milk.) Some doctors use bromocriptine to prevent lactation. The care of the woman after stillbirth requires sensitive attention to her physical needs to keep her as comfortable as possible, in addition to emotional considerations. Grieving may be delayed until the woman has recovered enough physical strength to address her loss.

Couples need to decide for themselves about burial and a memorial service for the child. To name the child and commemorate its death often help the couple grieve about a tangible loss and may mobilize their friends and relatives to offer comfort. Our society does not have rituals for comforting in miscarriage or stillbirth. Friends and relatives may not know what to do or say. All emphasis is on the future, "getting well," and "getting pregnant" again. The couple must defend their right to invent their own rituals to help them in the acknowledgment of a life begun and lost, and the grieving this deserves.

UNDERSTANDING WHY

When either a miscarriage or stillbirth occurs, the couple need to have some explanation about why it happened. If the miscarriage was early, the products of conception may have been lost in the blood flow. In a second-trimester miscarriage, there is a fetus of sufficient size to be examined by pathology. It is also important that the placenta be examined, as it may yield important information. In stillbirth, an autopsy is usually indicated. Because one of the concerns of a couple who have lost a pregnancy is whether to try to conceive again, this information is extremely valuable. If the problem was one not likely to occur again, the couple can proceed with that knowledge. If the pregnancy was lost for some reason that might recur but be treatable, the couple will enter into the next pregnancy under close monitoring. If the problem was a genetic disorder, further testing of the partners will reveal if future pregnancies might be at risk. In no case is it acceptable for a doctor to urge couples to "try again" repeatedly without the benefit of knowing what caused the pregnancy loss.

It is said that nature strives to complete a reaction. When a miscarriage or stillbirth occurs, a process has been stopped abruptly, never to be completed. Grieving focuses on that interruption and slowly builds a bridge to cross over it back to life. Some couples grieve but briefly; for others grief may be prolonged. Grief is experienced by each person and each couple in their own way at their own speed. It is common for feelings of loss to be reactivated at anniversaries such as the expected due date, the date of conception, and the time of the loss itself, perhaps for years to come.

> I still find myself thinking, if I were pregnant now, I would be seven months along. I already dread my due date in April. It will be spring then, and I would have been wonderfully expectant like all of nature.

8. New Technologies

First, do no harm.

HIPPOCRATES

*T*echnology has been defined as the application of science to solve problems. The problems of infertility have never been more accessible to technology, since for a given couple we now have an almost 90 percent chance of discovering the cause. The problem with science and its application is that research moves years ahead of social, legal, and ethical inquiry. While some scientists believe that any medical, surgical, or technical breakthrough deserves instant application, most would agree that medicine must exist in an ethical and legal framework that protects all parties involved. This, of course, takes time, and may involve a protracted social and political process as well.

Just because technology exists does not mean that it should be instantly available. However, people who might hope to benefit from the technology are often as eager as the researchers to make the leap from laboratory to life. Because of the intense motivation many infertile couples bring to their search for a baby, they are vulnerable to exploitation. Sometimes "informed consent" on the pros and cons of a technology proves very difficult because of the highly emotional and vulnerable state an infertile couple are in. This is of particular concern when for-profit programs outside of the major medical centers ascertain an unregulated situation for which there is a lucrative supply-and-demand market.

The new technologies of infertility challenge us all to further the aims of science and medicine while protecting the welfare of the people involved. Used carefully, these new procedures open up vast possibilities for treating previously hopeless cases. Used recklessly, technology could usher in the Brave New World of tomorrow. Ultimately, society will be the judge of the appropriateness of technology and whether persons have been helped or harmed.

IN VITRO FERTILIZATION (IVF)

There has been no more controversial method of applying technology to infertility than in vitro fertilization. When Louise Brown, the first "test tube baby" was born on July 24, 1978, in Oldham, England, it was the culmination of more than a decade of research by Drs. Robert Edwards and Patrick Steptoe. The first American baby by IVF was not born until 1981. The years leading up to this event illustrate the social and political nightmare that can result when a new technology is announced and greeted with social, religious, and ethical chaos.

In 1974 Dr. Pierre Soupart, a professor at Vanderbilt University, submitted an application to the National Institutes of Health (NIH) to fund a three-year study to determine the safety of human in vitro fertilization. In 1972 Soupart had been the first American to fertilize a human egg in vitro. His study proposed to fertilize eggs retrieved from volunteer women patients who were undergoing gynecological surgery for other reasons. These eggs were to be fertilized in a culture dish and grown up to six days to observe whether any abnormalities occurred, then disposed of. He did not intend to implant any fertilized embryos.

In the spring of 1975, NIH decided it would fund this proposal only after review by the Ethical Advisory Board (EAB) of the Department of Health, Education, and Welfare (HEW). Although a federal law created the EAB in 1975, it took two years for the government to appoint members and another six months for the EAB to begin its regional hearings. Secretary of HEW, Joseph Califano, charged the EAB with undertaking a massive fact-finding mission, not just reviewing Dr. Soupart's request, but making a broad analysis of all scientific, legal, ethical, social, and religious issues raised by in vitro fertilization. Ironically, just two months after these hearings began, Baby Louise was born in England.

The 15-member EAB was composed of physicians, medical ethicists, lawyers, civic leaders, and a psychiatrist. They worked from May 1978 to May 1979 holding hearings around the country and preparing their report. Testimony was received from medical and scientific experts, theologians, feminist groups (opposed), Right to Life activists (opposed), and infertile couples. RESOLVE was represented at each hearing by members who presented personal cases that could only be helped by the procedure of IVF.

After painstaking analysis, the EAB concluded that any broad prohibition of research involving human IVF was unwarranted in spite of the obvious recognition that this technology, as any other, could be abused. The most difficult decision of the board was regarding the moral status of an embryo. It concluded: "After much analysis and discussion regarding both scientific data and the moral status of the embryo . . . the embryo is entitled to profound respect, but this respect does not necessarily encompass the full legal and moral rights attributed to persons." Several conditions on the conduct of research provided that embryos not be sustained for more than 14 days after fertilization, and that the public be advised if the procedure resulted in abnormalities in offspring higher than those found in natural human reproduction.

In spite of the favorable ruling of the Ethical Advisory Board in May 1979, Secretary Califano took no further action on its recommendation. Pierre Soupart died in June 1981, never having received the grant he applied for seven years before. To this day no federal funds are available to researchers working in this vital area. In spite of this, with private funding Drs. Howard and Georgeanna Jones pioneered the first American IVF clinic at East Virginia Medical School. At the time of this book's publication, no fewer than 2,500 babies have been born of IVF and numerous clinics exist worldwide, about 200 of those in America.

The procedure involved in IVF varies slightly from clinic to clinic and is constantly being refined to increase the successful-pregnancy rate. Applicant couples are first screened to be sure they are candidates for IVF. Most clinics will not take women over thirty-five years because of increased risks of childbearing and genetic disorders and the poor rate of success. The couple should have exhausted all medical and surgical options, including the possibility of tubal surgery, before turning to IVF. The high expense (up to $5,000 per cycle) and the current low success rate (10 to 25 percent) should have been carefully explained. At this time, most insurance plans cover little if any of the expense of IVF. The couple should be screened for any infections, and the woman should have at least one normal ovary and a normal uterus. In vitro fertilization is most commonly used with couples who have been unable to conceive for reasons of blocked or absent fallopian tubes. Initially, IVF was used with couples who had normal ovulation and normal sperm counts. More recently, IVF has broadened in scope to include the possibility of donor semen and even donor eggs. Some clinics are using IVF successfully to achieve pregnancies in cases of low sperm counts, endometriosis, and even unexplained infertility of long duration.

The procedure begins with the woman being stimulated with an ovulation-inducing drug to be sure several follicles will ripen. Clinics use clomiphene citrate and Pergonal most commonly. The woman is monitored closely through blood levels for estrogen as a sign of follicular growth and ultrasound to see the number and size of follicles developing. When everything looks ready, HCG is given. The ripened eggs will usually be released within 38 to 42 hours after this injection. Laparoscopy or ultrasound-guided aspiration is used to harvest the ova before they are released. As many as 3 to 12 ova are collected.

Meanwhile the husband (or donor) brings a fresh semen specimen to the clinic. It is prepared by a process called sperm washing. Sperm washing involves separating sperm cells from seminal fluid by centrifuge. The sperm cells are then placed in a special medium, where the poor-quality sperm sink to the bottom and the more motile sperm swim to the top. These sperm cells are mixed with the collected ova 5 to 6 hours after the laparoscopy and allowed to incubate for 18 hours in a special medium. Fertilized eggs are located and transferred to another culture dish and medium to grow another 38 to 40 hours. At that time the fertilized eggs are examined to see if they are normal. They are usually transferred back to the woman at the eight-cell stage of development.

The woman is prepared for the transfer in a doctor's clinic or hospital setting. A soft plastic catheter is inserted into the cervix. Between one and four embryos are drawn up in a syringe with a nutrient solution and gently flushed into the woman's uterus via the catheter. She will generally recline for several hours to assist the embryo's implantation and then is discharged home. Some clinics recommend bed rest at home for a few days and abstinence from intercourse to further guard against pregnancy loss and assist implantation. Progesterone may be given if the woman's own levels are questionable to support pregnancy. An early pregnancy test may be done 10 to 14 days after the transfer to learn if implantation occurred.

The procedure just outlined represents the physical aspect of IVF but cannot begin to represent the emotional roller coaster that both couples and IVF staff experience while they wait to see if a cycle will be successful. Often the couple have come to IVF as a "last resort," having faced many procedures, expenses, and disappointments already. While they are advised of the low success rates, couples often choose not to hear this. It is imperative that a good IVF program have an experienced counselor who can prepare the couple beforehand and be available during procedures and afterward. Should the cycle be unsuccessful, the counselor needs to allow the couple to vent their grief and frustration and to offer helpful advice on what to do next. Most programs limit the number of cycles they will allow a couple to try; emotional and financial exhaustion may place a limit on how many times a couple is *able* to try.

The statistics on IVF vary from clinic to clinic, but most show similar ranges. The recovery rate for harvesting ripened eggs from the ovary appears to be about 90 percent. Superovulation with fertility drugs and close monitoring by ultrasound and blood levels are used to ripen multiple follicles and pinpoint the correct time for retrieval. Fertilization rates of eggs by sperm in vitro are also encouragingly high. However, birthrates range only about 10 to 20 percent. This is attributed to a variety of problems: poor fertilization; improperly timed transfers; inadequately prepared uterine lining; irritation of the uterine muscles during transfer, which may cause uterine contractions; improperly placed oocytes; disturbance of the cervical mucus plug; and higher risk of infection. Most in vitro research is aimed at solving these problems and improving the birthrate. *

If you are interested in learning more about in vitro and about clinics in your area that are accepting applications, RESOLVE has an up-to-date listing, which includes information on waiting periods and types of patients accepted.

GAMETE INTRAFALLOPIAN TRANSFER (GIFT)

GIFT is an acronym for *gamete intrafallopian transfer*. This involves placement of several ripened ova and a portion of a centrifuged semen specimen into the ampullary (distal flared portion) end of the fallopian tubes, which is thought to be the natural site of fertilization in humans. This is done during laparoscopy, at the time of the egg retrieval. GIFT is not an answer for women who have diseased or absent tubes, because it depends on tubal patency. However, it seems to have promise with couples who have unexplained infertility of long duration, in cases of low sperm counts, and in some stages of endometriosis.

The procedure begins with ovulation-inducing drugs to increase the number of ripening ova. Just before egg retrieval, semen is obtained from the husband. The semen is prepared by sperm washing, as with IVF. Ova are collected exactly as they are in IVF and examined for maturity and several are selected along with about 100,000 motile sperm and loaded into about 50 cc of medium in a syringe with a transfer catheter. The catheter is inserted through a laparoscopy incision and threaded 1½ to 2 cm into the ampulla of the tube. The procedure may be repeated on the other side.

The doctor who developed this technique, Dr. Ricardo H. Asch, has reported a 31 percent success rate in pregnancy with this technique. Although the sample of GIFT patients is small compared to IVF patients, it appears to have a considerably higher-term pregnancy rate. The greater success is thought to be due to the lower miscarriage rate since fertilization occurs in

---

* In vitro fertilization fact sheet, RESOLVE, Inc., p. 2.

vivo. In addition, this technique may be more cost-effective than IVF is, since it can be performed entirely during laparoscopy and does not require the large team of specialized technicians. Coverage by insurance is more likely than with IVF and the overall cost is much less. Disadvantages include the possibility of initiating a tubal pregnancy or inciting a tubal infection.

EMBRYO FREEZING

One problem of both IVF and GIFT is the possibility of multiple ova being fertilized or retrieved and the question of how many to implant in the woman without subjecting her to the risk of a large multiple gestation and its accompanying maternal and fetal risks. The use of cryopreservation to preserve human embryos can limit the number implanted while retaining embryos for use in future transfers should this attempt fail. It may also spare the woman a repeated laparoscopy and the expense of another cycle of treatment.

Scientists working in human embryo cryopreservation can learn much from animal husbandry, where the practice of freezing, thawing, and implanting embryos has gone on successfully for many years. The optimal stage for successful freezing seems to be the eight-cell embryo. A protectant fluid must surround the embryo to prevent the development of intracellular ice crystals. Embryos are frozen in liquid nitrogen in plastic straws by a computer-controlled biologic freezer. Both freezing and thawing must be accomplished in a slow, controlled process to prevent damage to the embryo.

The first infant born of a frozen embryo used in IVF occurred in 1984 in Australia. The number of IVF programs with capability for freezing embryos is still small but is expected to be an area of rapid increase as research and improvements in the technique develop. If successful, use of frozen embryos will reduce the cost of IVF when patients have to undergo repeated cycles.

Freezing of embryos seems to solve one ethical dilemma of IVF and create others. Activist groups have opposed IVF on several grounds, but none more strenuously than the "disposal" of extra embryos not needed in a given cycle. Recently the legal and ethical issues of human embryo storage and disposition of such embryos came into the news when an American couple who had flown to Australia for IVF were killed in a plane crash before they could use two embryos they had in storage. The options available were to donate the embryos to an unrelated couple, to donate them to an approved research program, or to dispose of them in accordance with hospital ethical standards. Clearly, a contract including use of frozen embryos should stipulate the fate of the embryos if the couple become unavailable for any reason.

Researchers foresee a time when egg banks may be as common as sperm banks, and one facility has already opened in New York. This would allow women to store their own eggs or fertilized embryos for use at a future time, or they could supply donor eggs or embryos to infertile women much as donor semen is now provided for infertile males in donor insemination.

EMBRYO TRANSFER

Embryo transfer (also called ovum transfer) is a new technology that has become available only recently for use in humans. This procedure also traces its roots to animal husbandry. Beginning as early as 1890, fertilized ova have been successfully transferred in more than 15 species of mammals. Each year tens of thousands of cattle are produced in this manner, with success rates of better than 60 percent (live newborns) per transfer attempt. It allows breeders to improve their stock by superovulating prize females and transferring these fertilized ova to common brood stock for gestation. Thus, a female that might have had 10 gestations in a normal lifetime might be able to provide 100 offspring instead. Animals such as sheep, which can carry twins easily, may be able to double their normal output.

Embryo transfer is a nonsurgical procedure appropriate for couples in which the woman is unable to produce ova or is worried about passing along a genetic disease. Candidates for the procedure might be women who have experienced premature ovarian failure, women who cannot be helped to ovulate with ovulation-inducing drugs, women with Turner's syndrome (congenital absence of ovaries), or women who have a genetic disease in their immediate families. The technique is also suitable for women with blocked or absent fallopian tubes or with unexplained infertility of long duration. The difference, in these last two cases, is that IVF would permit the woman to contribute her own ova, while embryo transfer relies on a fertile woman donor.

The steps involved in embryo transfer are quite simple: A donor is chosen who has been carefully screened for genetic history and who resembles the infertile woman physically and who has the same blood type. The donor is compensated with about $250 for each month she participates in the program. The donor and the infertile woman have to be "synchronized" in their cycles so they are within a day or two of each other. This can be done with use of birth control pills to delay the infertile woman in the cycle previous to the transfer cycle. If the woman has no ovarian function, natural hormone replacements accomplish this synchronizing of cycles. The donor is sometimes stimulated with ovulation-inducing drugs to ripen more than one follicle. With careful monitoring for the LH peak at ovulation time, the donor is then inseminated with sperm from the husband of the infertile woman.

Sperm are generally "washed" from the seminal fluid and selected for motility as in IVF. Fertilization takes place within the donor woman's fallopian tubes as in normal reproduction.

As with any naturally conceived pregnancy, the fertilized egg or eggs descend through the fallopian tubes and enter the uterus, where they float freely for about 5 days. A fertilized ovum does not implant in the uterine wall until the sixth or seventh day after ovulation. In embryo transfer, the free-floating eggs are harvested from the donor's uterus by means of a soft plastic catheter which is introduced through the cervix on the fifth day after fertilization. The uterus is lavaged with a special nutrient fluid, which is then drawn back into the catheter along with the ova. The entire procedure is painless and can be done in an office in a few minutes.

The recovered ova are examined microscopically. If cell division has taken place normally, the ova are immediately placed in a special transfer fluid and inserted into the patient's uterus through a catheter placed in the cervix. This too is virtually painless and can be done in the office. If an ovum implants, the patient will experience a natural pregnancy, even though she is "infertile."

The clinical availability of embryo transfer is still limited, but it is anticipated that its success rate will exceed that of IVF, while the cost per cycle is expected to be less than $3,000. Further, since this is a nonsurgical procedure, it can be repeated as many times as necessary. IVF is generally limited to four to six attempts. One obvious question the procedure raises is what would happen if all the fertilized ova were not harvested and the donor became pregnant, or if implantation had already taken place on the transfer day.

The major legal controversy surrounding embryo transfer is that the procedure was developed under financial sponsorship of a private corporation, which is seeking to patent the technique. Although other medical processes have been patented, embryo transfer may prove to be historical because of its commercial potential. Fertility and Genetics Research, Inc. (FGR) was formed in 1985. A public stock offering in December 1985 raised $3.6 million to fund the opening of the first FGR Ovum Transfer Centers. These centers may be likened to franchises of the corporation, which is in business to make a profit as a member of the stock market.

PART II

Psychosocial Aspects of Infertility

9. Mythological, Religious, and Social Influences on Fertility

Give me children or I die! . . .

RACHEL, GENESIS 30:1

At a time when achieving a high birthrate is no longer essential—in fact it's something of a concern in many countries—people continue to adhere to social, religious, and cultural values that tell them the destiny of each young man and woman is to marry and reproduce. Failure to reproduce, for whatever reasons, makes a couple suspect, targets of pressure and even ridicule, or objects of pity. It is important for infertile couples and those who deal with them to understand the history that has led to the present state of thinking about fertility and infertility.

From the earliest recordings of humankind there has been an obsession with fertility. Fertility of people and fertility of the land were necessary for survival, and the forces at play were thought to be one and the same. If the land prospered and bore fruit, so would its people flourish; a terrible drought would kill both plants and people. Because early humankind did not understand the natural phenomena that influenced life for better or worse, they developed mythological ways of thinking about them. This later gave way to more highly developed religious doctrines and societal codes. Thinking evolved from a primitive level to a sophisticated level in most matters, but many attitudes about fertility and infertility have remained in the realm of myths, taboos, and superstitions to the present.

MYTHOLOGY AND FERTILITY

A myth may be defined as a primitive view of the world that attempts to bring the unknown into relation with the known. The mythology of ancient Greece and Rome is filled with reverence for fertility, attributing enormous sexual potency and procreative powers to gods and great fecundity to goddesses. There were no less than four temples to Venus, the goddess of love, in Rome. Diana, goddess of the woods, was thought to help Romans achieve their families. Her counterpart in Greek mythology was Artemis, who was responsible for life in the woodlands. Artemis was revered as a goddess of fertility even though she was always portrayed as the "virgin huntress." A famous temple to Artemis was built in the Ionian city of Epheus, where she is represented as a many-breasted idol.

The cult of Venus (known in Greece as Aphrodite and in Syria as Astarte) required young girls to prostitute themselves. This practice was probably intended to increase the population as well as to provide servers for the temple. It is thought that this prostitution was also a way to test a young girl's fertility before she was given in marriage. Religious prostitution continued throughout the Middle East until the reign of the Christian emperor Constantine, who abolished the cult of Venus and ordered the temples destroyed.

An even older cult was the cult of Phallus. The penis or representations of it (phallic symbols) were revered as symbols of great fertility in as dissimilar cultures as those of India, Japan, Egypt, and Mexico. The phallus was usually represented as an enormous wooden penis and was carried in processions and worshipped in temples. In India, childless women would press their naked bodies against these giant fertility symbols in hopes of achieving pregnancy. In Egypt, women wore small porcelain phalli as amulets in hopes of increasing their fertility.

FERTILITY SYMBOLS AND RITES

Throughout history, symbols, rituals, and objects have been used or worshipped in the belief that they would promote fertility. Even after the influence of modern religions was felt, these pagan beliefs have persisted in many cultures.

One of the most common symbols of fertility in all cultures has been rain or water. As it was rain that brought productivity to the land, it was also thought to have a curative effect on a childless woman. Its symbol is the spiral, which is seen as very lucky and fertility enhancing. The sun is also a giver of productivity. It embodies the Chinese male yang principle, being hot and dry and active. Worship of the sun goes back to the earliest cultures. The moon, on the other hand, is very mysterious and female in its symbolism. The Chinese female yin principle is totally female, cool, moist, and passive. Crescent moons were particularly celebrated and thought to be auspicious symbols for fertility. In seafaring cultures fish were considered omens of fertility, as they were indeed the harvest that sustained life. Dolls were used to promote fertility in many ancient cultures, often worn or carried by a childless woman against her breasts or abdomen in the manner that a real child would be carried.

The rod, stick, staff, and scepter are all symbols of phallic power. The lingam, an ancient symbol for the transmission of life, was worshipped in India long before the Aryan invasion. The origin of the lingam was the digging stick or primitive plow, since both the plow and the phallus in their different ways prepare for insemination. *

The Jews believe that God breathed over still waters and started life into being. The Hindus believe that Shiva, lord of creation, danced and life was stirred into being. Life is movement and movement is life. Magic power was ascribed to circular motion. The ancient symbol of the swastika symbolizes the movement of the seasons. Turning clockwise, the swastika is life oriented and fertility granting. The action of sowing seed would always be from left to right. Turning counterclockwise, the swastika is life destroying and demonic. Ironically, Hitler used a clockwise swastika for the flag of the Nazi Third Reich on the advice of occultists. †

Certain plants and trees have been thought of as fertility symbols. The mandrake, also known as the "love apple," is mentioned in the book of Genesis as a fertility cure used by Leah. In East Africa the fig and banana trees were thought to be occupied by fertility spirits. In northern India and West Africa the coconut was given by priests to childless women. In Europe fertility has been associated with the maybush or hawthorn. In America rice is still thrown at the bride and groom as they leave on their honeymoon, a vestige of an old fertility custom.

RELIGIOUS INFLUENCE ON FERTILITY

The earliest worship in ancient communities of Asia Minor, Syria, and Libya was of a mother-goddess rather than of a father-god. Even though the man

---

* Pearl Binder, *Magic Symbols of the World* (London: The Hamlyn Publishing Group Limited, 1972), p. 23. A fascinating and thorough study of fertility symbols can be found in this book.

† Ibid., p. 23.

was stronger and more dominant, it was the woman who was the awe-inspiring mystery, with her monthly cycles corresponding to the cycles of the moon by which man first reckoned time in periods of more than one day. It was the woman who conceived, all alone or by some supernatural unseen power. (The discovery of spermatozoa in semen was not made until 1677 after the development of the microscope by Leeuwenhoek. The role of sperm in reproduction was not fully understood for another two centuries.) It was the woman who labored and gave birth and suckled and raised the young of the tribe. At some point man finally deduced that children were not conceived parthenogenetically—sired by a spirit of the wind or waters of the streams or the gods on high. From that time on the strength of worship of mother-goddesses declined, but it never really disappeared and was always connected with fertility of the land and of humans. Even today, a childless Catholic woman will pray to the Virgin Mary for assistance in conceiving a child.

In the book of Genesis, Adam and Eve were commanded to "be fruitful and multiply." In the early history of religions there was an enormous effort to multiply and produce children to make settlements and later to replace those men who died in battle, as tribe fought tribe. Most prized were boy children, as they would work the fields and tend the herds and be warriors. Girl children were valuable only in their potential to bear more children. The woman who was childless was as useless and despised as a piece of land that would yield no crops. The same word was given to both—barren. Practices later prohibited by religion, such as incest, adultery, polygamy, and religious prostitution, were excused as necessary to produce more children. Unproductive practices such as homosexuality, bestiality, and masturbation were thought to invoke mighty wrath from God. Abraham and Jacob were encouraged in the book of Genesis to beget children by their servants when their wives were childless.

> When Rachel saw that she bore Jacob no children . . . she said to Jacob, "Give me children or I die!" Jacob's anger was kindled against Rachel and he said, "Am I in the place of God, who was withheld from you the fruit of the womb?" Then she said, "Here is my maid Bilhah; go in to her, that she may bear upon my knees and even I may have children through her." (Genesis 30:1–3)

Five of the better-known childless women in the Bible, Sarah, Rachel, Leah, Hannah, and Elizabeth, all finally conceived through finding favor with God. Not only did they conceive, but they did so repeatedly, even at advanced ages, and most of the progeny were sons. In such religious recordings there is an obvious connection with fertility and worthiness. Infertility was a punishment meted out to those who lost favor with a vengeful God.

More recently, moral codes have been developed about sexual behavior and are reinforced by each major religion. St. Augustine was very influential when he proclaimed that intercourse, even with one's own lawful wife, was wicked and sinful if conception was in any way prevented. The Roman Catholic church remains adamant on this position even today. It not only prohibits birth control and abortion but also prohibits homosexuality, donor insemination, in vitro fertilization, and even masturbation. Orthodox Judaism takes an equally staunch position on most of these practices. Procreation took on an important value to those who viewed (and view) the pleasures of sex as sinful. One could take part in the sinful pleasure but feel vindicated only by an ensuing birth. *Motherhood purged sex.* It also purged women, who have been considered evil since Eve's first transgression.

> Adam was not deceived, the woman was deceived and became a transgressor. *Yet woman will be saved through bearing children.* (Timothy 2:14–15)

According to some religious teachings, children must be born in order for the woman to reach heaven, or to free souls from bondage, or to permit souls to go their way in a cycle of transmigrations. In some religions a marriage can be annulled if a woman proves infertile, although the reverse is not true if a man proves to be infertile. In polygamous marriages, an infertile wife is soon replaced by a new one and is often relegated to the level of servant. Large families have often been seen as a source of help and wealth, not only for the work they could do, but for the security they afforded to parents in their old age.

Religious influence over fertility and therefore infertility has been great in all religions past and present. It accounts for a large share of the attitudes displayed toward a couple who are childless.

SOCIETAL INFLUENCES ON FERTILITY AND INFERTILITY

Of all the forces that shape our modern attitudes and opinions, none can be stronger than the society we live in. Just as early humans devised myths to explain natural phenomena going on about them, so societies create myths and "traditions" to justify and perpetuate existing social patterns. Societal influences are really a combination of cultural, religious, racial, and socioeconomic factors. Therefore it is difficult (and unwise) to generalize about any such thing as "American society," embracing as it does so many variations. Some general trends are apparent, however, and their influence on fertility (and hence infertility) may be seen.

For generations, until the early 1900s, women had no access to birth control or abortion. The only logical role of the married woman was seen as childbearing and child rearing. Those exceptional women who varied from this pattern and chose careers often did so at the expense of marriage, as marriage would have forced them into childbearing. There were, no doubt, women who thought and worried about the injustice of having no right to make choices over their bodies, but their voices were few and far between until the early feminist movement. A brilliant essay, "Social Devices for Compelling Women to Bear and Rear Children," written in 1916 by Leta S. Hollingworth and published in the *American Journal of Sociology*, details some heretofore unthinkable thoughts by a woman:

> The fact is that child-bearing is in many respects analogous to the work of soldiers: it is necessary for tribal or national existence; it means great sacrifice of personal advantage; it involves danger and suffering, and in a certain percentage of cases, the actual loss of life. Thus we would expect that there would be a continuous social effort to insure the group-interest in respect to population, just as there is a continuous social effort to insure the defense of the nation in time of war. It is clear, indeed, that the social devices employed to get children born and that get soldiers slain, are in many respects similar.*

She debunks the myth that there exists such a thing as a "maternal instinct" that compels women voluntarily to seek the pain, inconvenience, and sacrifice of motherhood just to keep up the birthrate. She describes "social guardians" that protect motherhood and force women to conform to society's expectations. Among these guardians are public opinion, law, education, customs, art, and the tendency of society to value women on the basis of their fulfilling the maternal role.† As a point of interest, Ms. Hollingworth was married to a physician, became a clinical psychologist, and bore no children.

It is safe to say these "social guardians" are still in force today. We still hear about maternal instinct years after studies have proved that humans do not possess anything instinctive that makes them want children. What they do have is an innate desire for sex, and sex without birth control tends to produce children. What has been called instinct is really intricately learned roles and expectations from society. Public opinion is still largely favorable to motherhood and large families. Childfree couples are called "selfish" and "materialistic" by those who don't approve. Law, another social guardian, forbade legal use of birth control in some states until quite recently and forbade legal abortion until the momentous decision of *Wade* v. *Roe* in 1973. This latter right is a battle that is still being waged between the Right-to-Life movement on one side and the Pro-choice movement on the other. Education continues

---

* Quoted in Ellen Peck and Judith Senderowitz, *Pronatalism: The Myth of Mom and Apple Pie* (New York: Thomas Y. Crowell, 1974), pp. 19–20.

† Ibid., pp. 20–21.

in many ways to provide dual sets of roles, values, and opportunities to girls and boys. Much has already been said about customs and some of the religious and cultural practices that promote motherhood. Art is replete with "madonna and child" works which almost deify the state of mothering, adding to its mystique. Literature, too, is filled with references to childbearing as a coveted state. Sholom Aleichem's *Tevye's Daughters* offers an example:

> I don't want to boast, but all my daughters and daughters-in-law are fruitful, they all bear children every year. One has eleven, one has nine, another seven. Barren ones, that is, with no children at all, not one! Though with one son, the middle one, I had some difficulty. For a long time my daughter-in-law had no children at all. We wait and wait—not a sign of one. We tried everything. We went to doctors, rabbis. . . . We even tried a gypsy. Nothing helped.
>
> Finally there was only one thing left to do. He had to divorce her. Well and good, he'll divorce her. But when it came down to getting the divorce . . . Who . . . What . . . She didn't want it.
>
> "What do you mean, she doesn't want it?" I ask my son. And he tells me, "She loves me." "Fool!" I say. "Are you going to listen to that?" And he says, "But I love her, too." Now what do you think of that smart boy? I tell him *children* and he answers me *love*. What do you think of such an idiot?*

One area of influence on fertility (and therefore infertility) that cannot be overlooked is psychoanalytic psychology, which views parenthood as the *normal* outcome of development to adulthood. Freud, the father of psychoanalytic doctrine, had a negative view of female psychology in general. He believed that women were highly motivated to compensate for their lack of a penis (a state known as "penis envy") by having children. Freud believed that the only way a women could achieve a normal life was to accept her denuded condition and seek fulfillment through childbearing—ideally of male children, as they provide the longed-for penis. Freud's work has been subjected to review and criticism in recent decades and his ideas are not as totally accepted as they once were, However, updated versions of his essential message about women are found in the writings of Helene Deutsch, who undertook the massive two-volume study, *The Psychology of Women*, and also in the works of Erik Erikson.

That Freud made important contributions to the field of psychology is undebatable. But it is shocking how *totally* the Western World embraced his concepts for lack of any scientific evidence and passed them down to psychiatrists, psychologists, social workers, educators, doctors, nurses, and counselors. The same negative and prejudiced message about women was

---

* Sholom Aleichem, "The Joys of Parenthood," in *Tevye's Daughters*, trans. Frances Butwin (New York: Crown Publishers, 1949), pp. 109–10.

handed to the general public in popular magazines and journalism. The message, again, was:

> Little girls, from the moment they discover they do not possess a penis, develop an intense sense of envy and desire to have one. Since this is impossible, they grow up living in a state of castration and mutilation which can only be cured by the act of conceiving and bearing a child of their own.

When the first person (courageous soul!) said, "Hey! Girls don't envy boys because they have penises. Girls envy boys because they have all the power, privileges, and rights," a large chunk of "Freudian truth" suddenly looked very much like the Emperor's new clothes.

Pressure on couples to bear children comes from a combination of mythology, religion, culture, and society. Will such beliefs ever change? The answer, we hope, is yes. It is important to realize that institutions such as the family, society, and religion change very slowly. The effects of the Women's Movement, the availability of birth control, and concern with world overpopulation have begun to make changes in the thinking of people. Individual people change their ideas more quickly than the institutions they have created. We can hope for the day when each child born is a wanted child. And we can hope for the day that childless couples will be free from stigma and guilt.

10. Infertility as a Life Crisis

*What do we live for, if it is not to make
life less difficult for each other?*

GEORGE ELIOT
MIDDLEMARCH

*I*nfertility does not merely cause stress and anxiety to those affected. *It
represents a major life crisis.* In order to understand infertility as a life crisis,
it may be helpful to define the normal pattern of any event termed a *crisis*,
according to the work of Gerald Caplan:

1. A stressful event occurs that poses a problem that is insoluble in the
   immediate future.
2. The problem overtaxes the existing resources of the persons involved
   because it is beyond traditional problem-solving methods.
3. The problem is perceived as a threat to important life goals of the
   persons involved.
4. The crisis situation reawakens unsolved key problems from both the
   near and distant past.

INFERTILITY: A DEVELOPMENTAL CRISIS

There are many theories of the stages of growth and development of people.
In every theory there is a stage coinciding with young adulthood, marked by

101

the achievement of a sense of identity and maturity and a desire to create, procreate, or generate. One widely accepted theory of development is that of Erik Erikson. Erikson sees a person's lifetime as separated into eight basic ages and stages. Each successive stage builds on the last, and they progress to adulthood. It is implied in Erikson's theory that each stage can have either a successful or an unsuccessful outcome and that it is necessary to have a sucessful outcome to proceed onward to successful management of the next stage.

The stage of development of most interest when discussing infertility is that of *generativity*. Erikson describes generativity as "primarily the concern of establishing and guiding the next generation, although there are some individuals *who through misfortune or because of special and genuine gifts in other directions, do not apply this drive to their own offspring* [emphasis mine]."* The failure to achieve generativity leads to a state Erikson calls *stagnation*, or personal impoverishment. Another aspect of generativity is that all societal institutions—the family, schools, churches, government—safeguard and reinforce this behavior as desirable and codify the ethics of generative succession. Therefore, failure to reproduce may be seen as the failure to achieve an important developmental goal. Unsuccessful achievement of this stage denies the person progression to the final and most adult state of all, that of *ego integrity* (whose antithesis is *despair*). Whether or not one ascribes to the theories of Erikson, it is clear that infertility represents a developmental crisis.

MOTIVATIONS FOR PARENTHOOD

If infertility is accepted as a life crisis because it blocks the way to the life goal of parenthood, it might prove helpful to discuss some of the common motivations people have for wanting to become parents. *Not everyone wants to become a parent.* Childfree living is a trend that is acceptable and very much in vogue in some social strata. We are talking here about infertile people who have made the willful decision to become parents and then find they cannot. There are a number of motivating forces for parenthood.

Parenthood as a Way to Conform to Societal Pressure

Societal norms play a great part in the life goals people set for themselves. It is hoped that in the decades since Erikson formulated his theory, generativity

* Erik Erikson, *Childhood and Society* (New York: W. W. Norton and Co., Inc., 1950), p. 267.

has come to be recognized as having many forms besides the bearing and raising of children. But it is still true that society safeguards and reinforces all behavior relating to procreation and child rearing. Very large families are still seen by many as a signal accomplishment, even in this time of world overpopulation. Conversely, those who do not bear children, whether by choice or by accident of fate, are often prodded and provoked into revealing why they are not conforming to society's demand that married couples must produce offspring to be thought of as a "family." All institutions either subtly or blatantly press for conformity. If a couple is childfree by choice, the reaction is outrage. If the couple is childless by reason of infertility, the reaction is pity. Suggestions and advice are given unsolicited to both in hopes that they will succeed in bearing children and thereby become of value to society.

> One of my fears is that I'll die before I have any children and there will just be a tombstone saying "Mary Smith"—not "beloved mother of John and Sarah Smith." The more children you have, the more society values you. There was a terrible train-car collision in our town several months ago. A young married couple was killed. Their obituary was only several lines long and the caption read, "Childless Couple Killed." The message to me was that they were expendable since they had no children. And there was nothing much of value to say about them, because they had no children.

Parenthood as a "Rite of Passage" to Adulthood

In her excellent book, *The Growth and Development of Mothers*, Angela Barron McBride includes a chapter on why women (and men) have babies. She states:

> Having a child may mean that you are finally emancipated from your own parents. Once I was pregnant I expected them to see me as an equal, mature, no more their "flighty kid." Having the baby is a rite of transition. For a woman to be considered fully "grown up" in much of American Society, she has to have children. If she wants people to listen to her as a responsible person, she has to be able to show her credentials—Tom, Ann, Billy, Wendy, and so forth. *

There is much truth in this statement. Infertile people frequently relate stories of feeling like perpetual adolescents until they finally achieve parenthood by some means. This attitude seems particularly focused on the woman in the

* Angela Barron McBride, *The Growth and Development of Mothers* (New York: Harper & Row Publishers, 1973), p. 17.

couple. The man may show his credentials in other ways, most specifically in his education and his work. Many segments of society see a woman's education and work as something to do "until the babies come," and going back to work while children are very young still raises eyebrows, especially in the grandparent generation. The Women's Movement has been a vital force in legitimizing education and career as important aspects of any woman's credentials. ·

Parenthood as a "Reliving" of One's Own Childhood

In many couples there is a strong desire to bear and rear children in order to reexperience their own childhood through adult eyes. How often we hear poems and songs of the innocence and spontaneity of little children! The adult who witnesses such magic moments as a child running naked in a sprinkler, celebrating a first birthday, or welcoming the first family pet with open arms will remember his or her own childhood and be filled with nostalgia. If a person had a sad or impoverished childhood, he or she often desires to live vicariously through children and give them all the opportunities and joys that were missing from the previous set of parents. This, at times, can lead to difficult consequences for the child. People who truly desire a child as an extension of themselves are setting up a dangerous situation for the child, who must then be responsible not only for his or her own life, but for the parents' lives as well.

Parenthood as a Desire to Compete with One's Parents

In psychoanalytic theory much is made of wanting to bear children in order to compete with the same-sex parent. The man who produces a child is saying to his father, "See, I'm virile too." The woman is saying to her mother, "I'm a complete woman, like you." To have a smaller family may be a subtle way of saying, "See, we are smart about birth control and are not going to have more children than we can take care of." To have a larger family may be a way of saying, "We can handle *more* responsibility than you could." It is no doubt true that people wish to bear and rear children as a way of showing their parents they *can*. In cases where parents have been loved and admired, it is probable that the motivation is emulation rather than competition.

Parenthood as Role Fulfillment

The present generation in their childbearing years still have their roots most often in a traditional upbringing. The impact of feminism and antisexism regarding roles may not be felt for another generation, if then. Many young adults, however liberal, still define themselves in stereotyped male and female roles. The man expects to play his major role as impregnator of the woman, nurturer of the pregnant woman, and then provider for the young child or children. Provision means mainly bringing home a paycheck, and maybe some recreational time and occasional baby-tending on the side. The woman is much more involved in needing parenthood as role fulfillment. She may have formed her whole identity around the idea that she would one day marry and bear children. When this is denied her, she may feel totally "unemployed" even though she may work at a career she enjoys. She sees her identity as a woman as incomplete.

> When I was young and impressionable, I heard a neighbor of ours tell my mother that a woman was never truly complete until she conceived and bore a child. She certainly must have felt complete, since she had five children by three different husbands. I never questioned this idea. Later, when I was going through the worst part of my infertility struggle and conception looked hopeless, I learned that she had committed suicide, sitting in her car in a locked garage. And my first thought was—at least she died *complete!*

Another form of role fulfillment may be that imposed upon children by the parents. Some couples admit they wish to have children so they won't be "alone and lonely in old age." A supposition is made that one's adult children will be available and able to care for parents should infirmity or widowhood require it. That this often does not happen is in evidence all around us. It is not a healthy motive for parenthood.

Parenthood for Its Own Sake

Many people wish to bear and rear children because they actually *like* children! It has lately become fashionable to protest and despair over the rigors and sacrifices of child rearing, to say nothing of the expense. Infertile couples, unlike the general population, have two things going for them: First, they do not *have* to have children; quite the contrary, they have to work very hard to get them. Second, the months or years of effort involved in trying to achieve pregnancy or an alternative give the couple ample opportunity to review their needs and motivations for wanting children. That is not to say all infertile couples have healthy motivations or ultimately make the right decisions, just that they work very hard for what they get and they are usually very grateful for children and willing to take the rigors of parenting. This can lead to its own problems of feeling it is necessary to be a "superparent" or feeling guilty if the children ever complain. Parenting support groups for couples who have recently given birth or adopted can be very helpful in allowing the natural feelings of couples to be expressed in a supportive environment which helps them cope with the day-to-day responsibilities of raising a child or children.

MOTIVATIONS FOR WANTING A PREGNANCY

It is interesting that some infertile couples focus very much on the loss of the parenting experience, while others focus on the loss of the pregnancy experience. Many express desire for both the pregnancy and the end result, the child. There are a number of motivations for wanting a pregnancy.

Desire to Experience the Bodily Changes of Pregnancy

This feeling is naturally more profound in women than in their partners. There may be intense curiosity about what it would feel like to carry a baby inside, to swell and grow, to feel its kicks and movement, and finally to give birth. This state of pregnancy is often highly idealized, seen as an almost "holy" state, not the very real state of stretch marks, hemorrhoids, and heartburn it may be. Emphasis is placed on feelings of "glowing" and "blooming." When a woman says she wants to experience pregnancy to feel complete, she is actually saying *she wants to experience the total performance the body of a woman is capable of giving.* Her partner may wish to experience these feelings vicariously through her, as men in America are now more actively involved in pregnancy, labor, and delivery than ever before. Men often say they feel proud and virile in the presence of their pregnant mate. Women often feel "sexy." Pregnancy is a statement to the world that they are sexually attractive.

Desire for Genetic Continuity

"He's a chip off the old block!" carries the ring of genetic pride. Many people have great desire to see what their combined genetic material might produce. If the outcome is a handsome and bright child, they bask in the glory of what they have made. If the outcome is a sickly and dull child . . . well, there is always someone else in the family tree to blame for that. When there is a long line of succession in a family the situation may become extremely loaded if continuity is jeopardized. The last male child to carry the family name often feels undue pressure, not just to produce, but to produce a son. In some cultures women are divorced or succeeded by a new wife if they fail to produce sons, even though it is the male whose sperm determines the sex of a baby!

I married into the fourth generation of a family that came over on the *Mayflower*. After three attempts at pelvic and tubal surgery, and ultimately a hysterectomy, I now know I can never bear children. The pressure has been so great, my pain so intense that I offered my husband a divorce if he truly wanted one. Our marriage is not happy. I don't know what we will do. I think I know how Princess Soroya felt when she could not produce an heir for the Shah of Iran.

Pregnancy as Proof of Virility

In some cultures there is great machismo attached to keeping a woman constantly pregnant. In our culture, where discussion of sex is often explicit, people have other, more effective ways to allude to the success of their sexual relationships. In actual fact, pregnancy has a negative effect on the frequency and quality of sexual relations.

Pregnancy as a Narcissistic State

The love a woman has for herself (narcissism) may be invested in the fetus, and pregnancy may be experienced as an end in itself, not as a means to an end. In cases of neurotic narcissism, the woman desires not the child but the cherished state of pregnancy. Most women will confide that they feel "special" and a little pampered while in the pregnant state. The following quote describes some delightfully normal narcissistic thoughts:

> I do not ever want to stop being pregnant. My body enjoys a speeded-up metabolism. My pores have closed up, and my complexion is really rosy. I like to rest my hands on the jumping mound. I like to pat my stomach. I feel arrogant and wanton. . . . I am now too pregnant for sex. I feel virginal, precious. I am initiated into the sisterhood. . . . Who would ever have thought my whims would be accorded such importance. I have only to look a little winded and my husband does whatever I ask him to do. This is the first time in my life I've ever felt delicate or fragile. I never want to stop feeling precious. *

Pregnancy as Recapitulation of a Previous Pregnancy

For the woman who has lost pregnancies, either voluntarily by therapeutic abortion or by spontaneous abortion, the successful mastery of another pregnancy and labor and delivery may be extremely important.

---

* Angela Barron McBride, *The Growth and Development of Mothers* (New York: Harper & Row Publishers, 1973), p. 25.

I had an abortion when I was twenty. Who would ever have thought I would be infertile! After some months of trying, I finally had a pregnancy, but it ended in miscarriage. I was almost relieved, even as I grieved. I said, "God is getting even with me; now the score is even." But more problems developed, and it finally became clear there would be no more pregnancies. In my mind I keep going back to the pregnancies I had and trying to play them out to conclusion— but it is like a stuck record. I needed a successful pregnancy to complete what was interrupted. . . .

Desire to Breast-Feed

An aspect of pregnancy not to be overlooked is that it allows a woman to breast-feed her child. For an increasing number of young women in America, breast-feeding is enjoying a resurgence as a valued and healthful practice. Loss of the pregnancy experience also means loss of the breast-feeding experience. There are cases on record of women successfully nursing adopted children, but this is rare and involves unusual heroics to get a very minimal milk supply. It also requires adoption of an infant under 6 weeks of age.

My worst despair came over thoughts about breast-feeding—an experience I had always wanted. I bought a print of Picasso's *Mother and Child* and became very bitter at the thought I might not be able to duplicate that scene myself. Now that I have had a successful pregnancy I know I was right. Breast-feeding was an important and beautiful experience for me.

RESOLUTION OF THE CRISIS STATE

The Chinese symbol for crisis is formed of two words: *danger* and *opportunity*. The infertile couple who face a block in a cherished life goal are thrown into a state of crisis—a situation that their usual coping strategies cannot manage or solve. A period of emotional disequilibrium follows, which feels very dangerous. Crisis is associated with a rise in anxiety and tension, unpleasant and unfamiliar feelings, and a disorganization of ability to function as usual. It is a fact that people cannot stay in a state of crisis indefinitely, as it is too upsetting. Crisis is usually time-limited and pushes toward resolution within six weeks or less. The outcome may be one of three possibilities: The couple may emerge as stable as they were previous to the event; the couple may emerge with increased strength and emotional insight; or the couple may regress to a less stable level of functioning. This latter possibility is the reason all crisis states must be taken very seriously. The mental and physical health of the couple may ride on the outcome.

People in crisis are particularly vulnerable and can be gravely hurt by indifference among their family, friends, peers, or professionals working with them. The members of a couple often have very little help to give each other when they are in crisis together. Their feelings, which will be detailed in the following chapter, are confusing and exhausting and they are in a state of great turmoil, even though these feelings are normal and necessary to working through the crisis.

The positive side of this great vulnerability is that couples often seek help, in the form of a therapist, counselor, or support group at such a time. Since a state of crisis suspends the couple's usual coping mechanisms, they are especially open to learn new ways of coping. This can lead to new insights, changes in patterns, and tremendous growth. This is the "opportunity" of crisis. Since there is a rise in energy level in time of crisis, this energy can often be focused and directed by someone skilled in crisis intervention to help the couple move toward a positive resolution.

It is true of crisis that it may awaken key unsolved problems unrelated to infertility. For example, the person who never grieved over a parent's untimely death, may suddenly be overwhelmed with sadness for this loss as well as for the infertility. This is proof that events and feelings that are not dealt with directly do not "go away," but rather "go underground" and may become troublesome again and again until confronted. Therapeutic intervention allows an opportunity to deal with unsolved issues from the near or distant past as well as the current situation of infertility.

11. Common Feelings About Infertility

In our sleep, pain that cannot forget falls
drop by drop upon the heart and in our despair,
against our will, comes wisdom through the
aweful grace of God.

AESCHYLUS

*T*here are many complex feelings connected with infertility. Some of them are actual and rational, based on the very real and difficult events of investigation, attempted treatment, and decisions about alternatives. Other feelings are more irrational, based in part on myths and superstitions and on magical, childlike thinking about cause and effect. Whatever their origins, the feelings of infertility deserve to be studied in depth, both for the sake of the couple who feel no one else has ever felt the way they do, and for the sake of professionals who attempt to help them and find themselves unable to understand.

SURPRISE

No one expects to be infertile. The most common first feeling, though superficial and temporary, is one of surprise. People just naturally assume that they will be fertile if they decide to start a family. But couples cannot *know* they are fertile until they attempt to achieve a pregnancy. Many couples have used birth control for a number of years, waiting until everything in their lives was exactly right before beginning a family. Some couples have even agonized for years over *whether* to have a family.

How ironic for a couple to practice birth control for years and then discover a fertility problem existed all along. How ironic for a couple to question their desire or ability to parent and finally make the decision to do it, only to find the decision was not theirs to make!

DENIAL

"This can't happen to me!" How often people have hurled those puny words in the face of catastrophes and calamities that can and do happen to all of us. Denial serves a purpose. It allows the mind and body to adjust at their own pace to events that might otherwise be overwhelming. This is often true in a sudden diagnosis of absolute infertility, as in congenital absence of the vas in a man, or premature ovarian failure in the woman. Denial often comes into play at the time of miscarriage or stillbirth. The loss is too enormous to endure. It needs to be delayed a bit and then processed piecemeal until it can be fully absorbed. Denial is a protective defense mechanism which is appropriate to sudden and overwhelming events. It is not successful as a long-term defense mechanism, and it should break down in the face of reality to give way to the normal and necessary feelings to come.

ISOLATION

Even in this day of sexual candor, infertility is a personal and embarrassing subject to discuss. Much of this embarrassment has its roots in the superstitions and myths that surround infertility. If a couple choose to talk openly about their infertility, they open themselves up to gratuitous medical and psychiatric advice from all quarters: "Relax," "Take a second honeymoon," "Hang a maternity smock in your closet." Well-intentioned friends all have a name of a good doctor to recommend, and always stories of miracle babies conceived to others when all hope was lost. Much of this advice is directed, in whispers and behind closed doors, to the woman in the couple. The assumption is almost always made that the infertility problem resides with her.

With such attitudes abounding, it is not surprising that many infertile couples keep their problems carefully to themselves. This has two very unfortunate consequences. First, the family, friends, and peers of the couple may presume they are using birth control or do not desire children. This leads to needling and pressuring to start a family and fulfill society's dictates on procreation. Second, if the couple does not turn to others for support during infertility, they must, of necessity, turn to each other. This is often difficult, for they may be at different stages of feelings and one may be more motivated than the other to pursue treatment or alternatives. More significant, one is a man and one is a woman. The woman may have difficulty describing her despair over getting a period to one who has never menstruated. The man may be unable to communicate his feelings over "sex on demand" to one who has to have neither an erection nor an orgasm during intercourse.

> The husband I always thought would be there to stand by me turned away. After all, he's not a woman. He's not the one the doctor is examining under a microscope. His life hasn't really changed. Even if I did have kids, his routine would be basically the same. Because he's not the one going through all the tests he can't be faulted for not understanding when I dissolve each time my period comes. I blame myself for not being able to make him understand my pain. And then I feel angry. Why *can't* he understand?

Another form of isolation comes as the couple attempt to protect themselves from social gatherings and events they know will be painful. It is very common for an infertile couple to become highly sensitized to pregnant people and to baby announcements and christenings, yet it may be seen as socially mandatory to attend christenings, to ask to hold a new baby, to buy gifts and send cards. These social amenities become excruciatingly painful for a time.

> My dearest friend got pregnant and asked me to be godmother when the baby was born. I cried when I got home—for me. I wanted it to be *me* having the baby. I was jealous. . . . I'd tried harder, waited longer. I deserved it so much! Then I thought—am I so small and selfish that I've lost the ability to love and be happy for the people I care so much about? Oh God, what's happened to me!

Sometimes the infertile couple will radically change their life-style to avoid the painful reminders of others' fertility. This may lead either partner to quit a job that involves children, move from a neighborhood of families to one without children, and cut off ties with married friends who have children. The isolation may become extreme, until it feels as if there is no one else in the world who has ever been infertile and, conversely, as if fertility is everywhere.

> I remember going to the supermarket one night and being assaulted by the fertile world. At the bubble-gum machine, a mother was helping her toddler put a penny in the slot. A bit further down the aisle I was passed by a woman balancing a quart of milk and four containers of yogurt on her protruding belly. At the bakery one woman shouted across the buns to a young man, "Was it a

boy or a girl?" It is an unwritten law that what you want most seems to elude you but no one else. The gnawing desire to become pregnant is accentuated by every young mother or pregnant woman you see. And take my word for it—they are everywhere. . . .

ANGER

When a couple enter into investigation and attempted treatment of their infertility they surrender much of their sense of control over their bodies and destinies. Even in the best of medical relationships it is possible for extreme helplessness to be felt. The reaction to loss of control and helplessness is often anger.

> There is no inner recess of me left unexplored, unprobed, unmolested. It occurs to me when we have sex that what used to be beautiful and very private is now degraded and terribly public. I bring my charts to the doctor like a child bringing a report card. Tell me, did I pass? Did I ovulate? Did I have sex at all the right times as you instructed me?

> Never have I met a barrier I couldn't actively deal with. If it meant studying more or tackling harder, there was something I could do to improve myself. Work harder! Work longer! Eventually everything succumbed. But I can do nothing to make my sperm more numerous, more motile. Nothing!

The anger may be very rational, focused at real and correctly perceived insults, such as pressure from family to "produce" or the pain and inconvenience of various tests and treatments. Sometimes the anger is more irrational and may be projected onto targets such as the doctor, a certain relative, or an adoption worker, if the couple is exploring that alternative.

The real target of anger in either case is both the situation and the self. A "situation" is too diffuse to attack. To attack oneself is painful beyond bearing. Defense mechanisms rush to protect the self. The result may be the projection of anger onto authority figures, or onto relatives, or even onto an innocent and beloved fellow sufferer, the marriage partner. Anger that isn't acknowledged or released is often repressed and may lead to chronic depression. Feelings this powerful will not "go away" if we just ignore them. They will wait around indefinitely and become troublesome at some point. It is only a matter of time. One of the best ways couples have found to release their anger without detriment to themselves or others is through therapy or a support group. (RESOLVE support groups are offered in most states.) There a person can be honest with his or her feelings. Anger can be expressed and ventilated. Anger dissipates in the telling (and retelling) of the offending situation.

Because many people view anger as a socially negative feeling, it helps to find a "safe place" in which to express it.

Decisions that might be relatively simple to other couples become very difficult for infertile couples. Should they live in an apartment or buy a new house in the suburbs? Can they justify owning a house with no children? Should they take a new job offer even though it means relocating and leaving their infertility specialist? Should they save money for the future or spend and enjoy in the present? Should one of them take a business trip during their "fertile days?" Decisions to continue education or change careers are particularly hard for a woman who does not know when, if ever, she may get pregnant and have to take time off. All aspects of life become complicated by infertility and the result is predictable—anger.

GUILT AND UNWORTHINESS

It is logical for people to try to make a cause-and-effect relationship between infertility and something they have done (or not done) in life. All people can think of something to feel guilty about if they review their lives thoroughly. Infertile people frequently decide that they are not being blessed with a pregnancy because they are in some way *unworthy*. Just as in the Bible, pregnancy is being withheld as a punishment. The event that precipitates guilty feelings and thoughts of unworthiness may be amorphous, such as "not being a good person," or it may be grounded in real events. Some common guilt producers are premarital sex, an abortion, use of birth control, sexually transmitted disease, a previous divorce, masturbation, homosexual thoughts or acts, and even sexual pleasure. Fertile people may experience any or all of these situations and never feel a pang of guilt. The infertile person may draw a direct cause-and-effect conclusion.

Once the guilty act is acknowledged, the infertile person goes through a stage of bargaining or atoning, with fate or God, so that the guilty act may be forgiven and the punishment ended.

> Giving blood is painful for me; the veins collapse and go into spasms, and sometimes it takes 10 or 15 minutes of probing to get a sample. But in the months after my diagnosis, when blood was being drawn regularly to double-check my FSH levels, I welcomed the pain. The longer it took to find a vein, the more it hurt, the bigger the black-and-blue mark, the better! I bargained constantly with fate: a year of my life, ten years, my right arm, *anything* in exchange for a pregnancy. It seemed to me there was no amount of pain I wouldn't gladly undergo in exchange for a body that could make a baby. Maybe that's what fertility rites and ritual sacrifice are all about. I'm an educated

woman of the twentieth century, but emotionally I guess I'm not much different from my cave-dwelling ancestors. Rationally, I don't believe in their gods—but I still bargained with them, offering sacrificial blood samples.

When the prayers, sacrifices, and atonements of the infertile person go unheeded, more anger is often experienced at the *injustice* of the way fertility is dispensed. On the one hand are seen abortions, abandoned and battered children, people saying they wish they had never had their children; on the other hand, people are longing for children. Anger is felt toward God or life or fate that such injustice can exist.

> I began to volunteer in the local Children's Hospital. I loved holding the infants and mothering them and cuddling them. It tore my heart up to see the kids without visitors the whole time I was there. Here I am filled with love and caring for strangers. Their own parents cannot even find the time to visit.

This theme can be extended to the point where a person feels there is no point in working toward excellence or worthiness in anything. Jobs, education, even marriage may suffer the consequences if a person decides there is no point in trying to be worthy any longer. Indulgence in self-destructive habits such as drugs, excessive alcohol, and total apathy toward life may result. Most often the feelings of guilt and unworthiness are happily worked through in a support group or therapy situation that stresses several important points: First, people do not control all aspects of life, however much they would like to; second, life is not always fair; finally, worthiness and fertility are not related.

> I finally got to the point where I realized that pregnancy is not a reward for worthiness. Worthiness is its own reward.

DEPRESSION

The feeling of depression can be seen in two distinctly different mechanisms in infertility (and probably in any other crisis). *Pathological depression* is a smoke screen behind which some much more powerful and frightening feelings lurk. Inability to address denial, anger, guilt, or grief can lead to repression of these natural and necessary feelings. A chronic depression can ensue that may continue indefinitely until the real feelings are acknowledged. More will be said of this form of depression in discussion of unsuccessful resolution of feelings.

Normal depression is a real and legitimate state of sadness, despair, lethargy, and vague symptoms of distress. It is a natural phase of moving from anger and rage to the acceptance that a loss has occurred and that grief is imminent. When infertility is marked by an end point—a final diagnosis—depression will quickly give way to grief. One might describe the depression stage as a sort of "doomed" feeling, a subdued pregrief state. When infertility is not conclusive, but the couple are caught up in attempts at treatment which may be statistically uncertain, each cycle may go through a roller coaster of hoping and despair until they either are successful or cannot endure the pain any longer. Some couples never even get an answer to why they are infertile so that no treatment can be prescribed. These couples are very likely to have long depressive states, as they are never really free to grieve.

GRIEF

When a final diagnosis is reached that pregnancy will be impossible, or if a couple truly give up the quest for pregnancy of their own volition, the feeling that is necessary and unavoidable is *grief*. The grief is for the loss of a life goal, the loss of fertility, the loss of children who might have been born, and the loss of the pregnancy experience itself.

> Death. Death of a lot of things. The end of our family and our family name. It dies with us, because of me. My husband is the last male child in his family. Death before life. . . . before we even knew our child, because he never existed. The hardest part of this kind of death is the fact that it is the death of a dream. There are no solid memories, no pictures, no things to remember. You can't remember your child's blond hair or brown eyes, or his favorite toys or the way he laughed. Or the way it felt to be pregnant with him. He never existed.

It is a strange and puzzling kind of grief. The rituals society has for death pertain to actual losses, not potential losses. There is no funeral, no wake, no burial, no grave to lay flowers on. And friends and family may never even know. The couple often grieve alone.

It is well and good to talk of a "couple" but when infertility is confirmed and rests solely with one partner, that person stands alone for a time and realizes both the very personal loss and the fact that this loss denies genetic children to the other partner as well. The infertile person may entertain fears or fantasies that the fertile partner will leave—or worse, will stay and be secretly hostile and condemning. Many couples have problems verbalizing this concern. The fears may lead to a sort of self-fulfilling prophecy. The infertile partner may behave erratically or angrily in an attempt to goad the other partner into actually leaving or (in most cases) into revealing the dreaded negative feelings about the infertility. This should not be confused with laying blame, as infertility is a blameless event. But it *is* necessary for the fertile partner to be allowed to express feelings of sadness, disappointment, and grief along with the infertile partner. Expressions of unwavering love, fidelity, and "I never wanted kids anyway" seem to hurt the infertile partner and produce more guilt than the actual admission of honest feelings.

> He was so loyal, so accepting, so totally loving, that I could not believe I was seeing his true reaction. I had dreams of his divorcing me or coming home to tell me he had gotten another woman pregnant. There followed a time when I drank excessively and behaved outrageously. I picked on him, I clobbered him with every physical and social defect I could find in him. We now, laughingly, refer to these as my "Virginia Woolf routines." Anyway, one night I finally got him to cry and made him admit that I had let him down by not bearing him children—and that he was actually sad that he would never see his own genetic children. He let me know I had put him through hell to get to the point of this admission. He had not wanted to hurt me, he said. I told him I could live far easier with his sadness and depression than all that love. It was a definite turning point in our ability to accept what had happened to us.

The Course of Normal Grief

Grief that is experienced runs a very predictable, classic course. It is helpful to point this out to those who are grieving and those who want to help them. One of the most frequently heard reasons for *not* grieving is the fear that if one ever gives in to the feelings and tears, grief will be like a bottomless pit and one will never be able to stop.

The first stage of normal grief is frequently shock and disbelief. This is analogous to denial and allows the couple to absorb a loss gradually so that they will not feel overwhelmed. Infertility often unfolds in gradual fashion, with increasing loss of hope as the final diagnosis nears. Shock is most often seen when the couple experiences a sudden, unpredictable, and final event.

> We found out about my infertility almost by accident, long before we actually considered starting a family. It came in one blow, one sentence from the doctor—no uncertainty, no use for more tests, nothing more to be said. In a way we were strangely cheated. We never had a chance to make the happy decision, "Let's have a baby." My fertile years were over before they began. The loss was somehow unreal, confusing, because it was a loss not of something concrete, but of something potential. When my father died suddenly in the night, twenty years ago, I remember that for months afterward his death seemed unreal. I'd wake up every morning thinking: "Nothing has really happened. I dreamed the whole thing. I'll go into my parents' room and find them both

there." I experienced the same confusion with my infertility. It felt like a bad dream. Nothing had changed in my everyday life: No one had died, no one was sick, everyone looked the same. *Yet everything had changed.*

The second stage of grief is actual suffering—experiencing the painful feelings of sadness and emptiness. This stage is often accompanied by weeping and sobbing, and the physical symptoms of loss of appetite, exhaustion, choking or tightness in the throat, and sighing. The loss and feelings about the loss are reviewed over and over, often in waves of alternative active and passive states. This "griefwork" progresses, and the acute stage of suffering will generally pass within several weeks to several months. It seems to pass most quickly to those who "give themselves up" to the work of grieving.

Finally the third stage of grief, recovery, begins. Signs that the grieving couple have successfully freed themselves from ties to the lost object begin to be seen. The couple wish again to establish relationships and new interests; they try to function as they did before the loss; and they show renewed ability to experience pleasure, diversion, and satisfaction. Grief, of course, may be reactivated from time to time as the couple have reminders of their loss. But the suffering is never as acute again. Anniversaries of losses, holiday times, and family get-togethers are often difficult times. In infertility, other couples' pregnancies and births, christenings, and any reminder of babies in general may reawaken the loss.

Why Grief May Fail

The loss of fertility, the loss of a life's goal, the loss of children and the pregnancy experience—all are certainly of sufficient magnitude to require grief. Why is it then that one of the most common situations encountered in infertility counseling or support groups is that *no grief has taken place?* There are a number of very understandable and logical deterrents to normal grieving in infertility:*

1. *There may be no recognized loss.* A very real barrier to grieving occurs when the couple do not recognize the losses they have experienced. As has been mentioned, it is often the loss of a *potential* not *actual* object. Friends and family are frequently not aware of the infertility problem, and hence they do not offer support. Loss in miscarriage or stillbirth, although tragic, is more conducive to normal griefwork, as it is the loss

---

* For a number of the concepts under "Why Grief May Fail," the author acknowledges the excellent contribution to the subject of bereavement by Dr. Aaron Lazare in *Community Mental Health and Target Populations* (Englewood Cliffs, N.J.: Prentice-Hall, Inc., 1976).

of an actual child and family and friends are more often aware and able to be of support.

2. *There may be a "socially unspeakable" loss.* Some losses are difficult for members of the social support system to address. Both male and female infertility are laden with sexual overtones and embarrassing for some people to discuss. Even those who would like to come to the aid of the couple may feel the subject is too "private" or "better left alone." Other examples of unspeakable losses in society include hysterectomy, abortion, divorce, and disfiguring surgeries (amputations, colostomy, mastectomy, and so forth).

3. *There may be uncertainty over the loss.* In cases where infertility does not come to a conclusion, there is an element of uncertainty over whether there has, in fact, been a loss. Some people have likened it to the feeling of having a loved one missing in action in war. Possible loss is not actual loss. Both the couple and their family and friends do not know how or when to deal with the situation. It may not be until the woman comes to the end of her childbearing years in menopause that the couple actually give up hope and begin to grieve.

4. *There may be social negation of the loss.* There are some events, including infertility, that may be socially negated as a loss. Some people simply do not understand the devastation of infertility to a couple who want children. They are quick to point out, "You can always adopt!" (as if it were that easy) or they negate the value of children by saying, "You don't know how lucky you are!" Others compare infertility with life-threatening health conditions and tell the couple, "Be glad it isn't cancer." Needless to say, the couple are not comforted by these remarks.

5. *There may be absence of a social support system.* Because the griefwork of infertility is intense and painful, there may be great reluctance to give in to it in the absence of family or friends who can give comfort. We are increasingly a society without roots—more than 30 percent of our population moves every year. Loved ones may be far away when the need to grieve arises. Some people who are isolated from friends and relatives are able to seek out professional help in the form of therapists, counselors, or support groups to comfort them in the lonely task of grieving.

RESOLUTION OF THE FEELINGS OF INFERTILITY

Resolution may be defined as working through a difficult feeling or emotion. There are three distinct steps in achieving resolution: (1) The particular feeling is discovered and named ("This is anger that I am feeling"); (2) the named feeling is talked about as honestly as possible and the origins of the feeling are discovered and "worked through"; and (3) the person feels relief from and subsiding of the bothersome feeling and is ready to progress to a new feeling state. An impediment in the normal course of resolution is termed a *block*.

Unsuccessful Resolution

If a person experiences a block in any of the major feelings about infertility, progress in resolution is halted. A block may be brief or it may exist for a prolonged period of time. Usually it is caused by factors in the actual situation as well as by a failure of coping mechanisms.

A block in the feeling of denial is uncommon, but also perhaps the most serious and difficult to help. For some people self-esteem and sexuality are extremely threatened by admission of an infertility problem. It seems better to leave matters inconclusive than to have an absolute diagnosis. It may be that the person has a marginal commitment to the marriage or to parenting. It may be that total communication breakdown has occurred within the couple. If one member of the couple is denying heavily, it is almost impossible for the other member to progress. This kind of couple usually does not proceed with infertility investigation or may reject a diagnosis and "shop" from doctor to doctor for a more favorable one. They rarely enter into treatment because that would require admitting someone is infertile. They often cannot refer to themselves as *infertile* and are reluctant to discuss their situation with anyone. The problem with denial, as we have said, is that it doesn't work. It is intended to be a coping mechanism of short duration that eases a person into gradual acceptance of the problem. It is not intended to be a solution to the problem. Because denial involves pretending the problem just doesn't exist, enormous energy is required to maintain this state in the face of reality.

A block in the feeling of anger is quite common and may be understandable in certain situations. It may be seen, for example, in the couple who have been woefully mismanaged by a doctor or series of doctors and whose investigation and treatment is very protracted. Likely candidates for a block in the feeling of anger are those who are highly achievement oriented and those who believe steadfastly that they have absolute control over the course of their lives. The block can occur in one of two ways: Some people see angry feelings as very socially negative and therefore never address their angry feelings at all. Others may be able to name and confront the feelings of anger, but they get caught in a merry-go-round of effort aimed at reacting to the situation instead of accepting it. Such people are in such perpetual outrage that they cannot control their lives as they wish. Rage is hard to bear when it is directed inward, so it is often projected onto authority figures such as doctors, nurses, counselors, or adoption workers, or onto a selected relative, friend, or the marriage partner.

A block may occur in the feelings of guilt and unworthiness. People who are fatalists or those who have very low self-esteem are particularly vulnerable. They accept without question that infertility must be caused by "something I did wrong." They believe in their hearts that they are not worthy, and they keep their guilty feelings very secret for fear anyone else might find out how "bad" they are. As an attempt to bargain or atone for all this "badness," such a person may wage campaigns that are masochistic in order to be delivered from the punishment of infertility. It is interesting how often the atoning takes the form of volunteer or paid work with unwed mothers, work in pediatrics, child care, maternity, crisis counseling, or abortion clinics. Such proximity to sensitive areas can only be excruciating to the infertile person.

A block in grief may occur for the many reasons already mentioned, and it is the most common block of all in the steps toward resolution. It is also the easiest and most gratifying to help. Frequently all the couple need to facilitate their grief is: (1) permission to grieve; (2) understanding that a loss of great magnitude has taken place and that grief is normal; (3) a support system to comfort them as they grieve; and (4) awareness that grief runs a predictable course, and that it will end and recovery will follow.

A block in any of the important feelings of infertility can lead to the state previously described as chronic pathological depression. The symptoms that are presented are similar to those seen in normal depression—sadness, fatigue, vague physical symptoms, anxiety, restlessness. These distressing symptoms may bring the person or couple to therapy or counseling in search of relief. The counselor first establishes trust. The person may be so blocked that he or she does not even recognize infertility as a precipitating event for the depression. Slowly the story will unfold, and sooner or later will be seen a feeling that is so painful, so incapacitating that the person cannot address it or work it through. With careful perseverance, the counselor can help the person discover the feeling and its origins and begin to discuss it and overcome it. Only then can the process of resolution progress.

> I realize all of this was natural. I *had* to go through it. I *had* to work it all out and come to terms with myself. I had to face my feelings and reactions before I could go on. I had to make new life goals. I had to face the grief, the frustration, the hurt, the anger. I had to ride it through until it was over. These are normal, natural feelings. I am still working them out. . . . Maybe it's a lifetime thing and I'll never overcome it. All I know is I'm working on it, and that's what counts.

Successful Resolution

In successful resolution, each of the feelings detailed in this chapter is addressed, experienced, and overcome. That is not to say the feelings are laid to rest forever. Events may from time to time trigger the feelings anew and require that they be acknowledged and handled again. Each person probably has one feeling to which he or she is particularly vulnerable; for one it may be anger, for another guilt or grief. It is helpful to understand one's areas of vulnerability and to make a wry, "That's the way I am" acceptance of it. Some people recycle through their feelings about infertility so many times that they despair whether they will *ever* be able to get beyond them. *Such is the strength of these feelings.*

Finally, one day, a point of acceptance is reached where a couple conclude that they can put the active thoughts of infertility behind them, make some alternate plans, and get on with life. The ideal process of the stages of resolution might be modeled after Elisabeth Kübler-Ross's "stages of dying."* What do infertility and dying have in common? Perhaps more than one would expect. Here is a brief summary of the five stages:

1. Denial—"No, not me!"
2. Rage and anger—"Why me?"
3. Bargaining—"Yes, me, but . . ." (analogous to guilt)
4. Depression—"Yes, me." (analogous to grief)
5. Acceptance—"Yes, me, and I can accept it."

Successful resolution is characterized by a return of basic faith and optimism and a desire to turn energy previously caught up in infertility problems into new endeavors. The couple accept the obstacle in their life goals and find a way around it. The decision is made to do something alternative, such as to adopt a child or to try donor insemination or to remain childfree. Not only do they discuss the alternative (which happens very early in some infertility cases), they are now ready to act on it with confidence and optimism. People who have successfully resolved their infertility can usually talk of their crisis without weeping or becoming upset. There is more a sense of "sweet sadness" than the former bitterness.

My infertility resides in my heart as an old friend. I do not hear from it for weeks at a time, and then, a moment, a thought, a baby announcement, or some such thing, and I will feel the tug—maybe even be sad or shed a few tears. And I think, "There's my old friend." It will always be a part of me. . . .

12. Sexuality and Infertility

> . . . *and first I put my arms around him yes*
> *and drew him down to me so he could feel*
> *my breasts all perfume yes and his heart*
> *was going like mad and yes I said yes I*
> *will Yes.*

> JAMES JOYCE
> ULYSSES

It may be a quantum leap from the romantic passion of Molly Bloom to the bedroom of the infertile couple. When one partner implies, "Tonight's the night," the answer may be, "No I won't, no I won't. No."

The impact of infertility on sexual relations, sexual pleasure, and sexuality in general for many couples is so important that it deserves separate discussion from other feelings. It is important to qualify this chapter at the outset by saying: (1) sexual dysfunction or problems is *not* a significant *cause* of infertility, but rather an adverse *effect* of some situations, and (2) not all couples experience distress in their sexual relations while dealing with infertility. However, infertility counselors, doctors, and nurses are aware that for a great number of couples sexual relations that were once pleasureful, romantic, spontaneous, and orgasmic, may be reduced for a time to an act as perfunctory and uninspiring as brushing one's teeth.

PROBLEMS DURING INVESTIGATION AND TREATMENT

One of the first steps in the infertility investigation is the keeping of a basal temperature chart. This chart is important, as it serves to indicate whether ovulation appears to be taking place and, if so, when. The doctor usually points out the best "fertile time" as seen on previous charts and instructs the couple to have sexual relations on alternate nights around that time. Many doctors send the couple off with a cheery admonishment not to let charts "ruin their sex lives." But the couples are intent on doing exactly what they have been told. They follow their instructions to the letter. They may, at first, feel a sense of purpose of "mission" as they embark on programmed sex and plotting little X's on the graph. This sense of dedication is generally short-lived.

Three in the Bed, or the Ménage à Trois

A man, a woman, and a thermometer make strange bedfellows. The act of charting each day of the menstrual cycle and each sexual encounter focuses attention morbidly on infertility and the attempt to overcome it. Converting sexual relations to little X's on a chart also makes public something that most couples consider very private and do not ordinarily keep a running scorecard on.

> We felt like we always had someone between the sheets with us. First and foremost there was the thermometer. Then the doctor. We felt at various times as if both sets of our parents were in the bed with us. And, finally, during adoption, the social worker seemed to join us in the bed. During this whole time we never had that bed to ourselves!

There seem to be problems no matter *who* does the charting and who reminds the other that the fertile time is approaching. Trouble most often brews when one member is taking sole responsibility for keeping the chart and the other does not feel any responsibility to participate.

> As the infertility problem was mine, I took full charge of the temperature charts. When the fertile time approached, I could feel myself getting more and more anxious and angry inside. Ordinarily my husband was the instigator of sex. During my fertile time I felt I had to *seduce* him. What often happened was that we ended up fighting instead of making love. Then I would cry and tell him he didn't love me or want us to have a baby. And he would storm around saying he was no "goddamn stud service." Finally I realized what was happening. I took the chart and taped it to the headboard of our bed and showed him how to interpret it. I told him it was up to him to let me know when he wanted to make love. That worked much better.

The intrusion the basal temperature chart makes into a living pattern may also be painful. The instructions may ask that couples attempt to get the same amount of sleep each night, take the temperature at the same time each morning, note any ingestion of alcohol, and so forth. It must be remembered that charting is a crude tool at best. Attempts at fine tuning it by imposing additional restrictions on couples make no sense and are bound to add to an already frustrating experience.

Mental Charting

Ordinarily the doctor has a woman chart her cycles only as long as necessary to determine ovulation patterns and to schedule the initial tests. When this has been accomplished, charts are no longer necessary, except for certain treatments (AIH, in vitro, AID). Instead the doctor generally advises the couple to have sexual relations alternate nights around suspected ovulation, and sooner or later they will hit the right time if both have no other fertility problem. It is hard to explain to doctors that *couples don't stop charting just because they are not writing things down*. They just transfer the charting to a mental level. Ask any woman who is infertile and not charting anymore what day of the cycle she is in and she can tell you. Ask any couple when they must have sexual relations and they can tell you as unfailingly as if the chart were taped to their headboard. This mental charting may continue indefinitely and may be a source of stress the couple is not even aware of. The woman is the more likely one to be counting, as she is the cyclic one, the one who ovulates, the one who menstruates. Anxiety, depression, and fighting over sex can often be traced to this source. Counselors often recommend "holidays" from the quest for pregnancy to relieve this stress. Some couples will go so far as to use condoms or a diaphragm to stop thinking about conception.

Frequency of Relations

Most couples, infertile and otherwise, fantasize about how often other people have sex. They generally feel that others probably have more sex than they do and that they may enjoy it more.

> One way the temperature charts really hurt us was in the frequency with which we felt we had to have sex. I guess neither of us was that eager for sex 3 or 4 times a week. We both worked, we were both tired a lot, we had both had active sex lives prior to marriage (see, I'm defending us even now). The ultimate moment for me was when I found myself "cheating" on the charts. I put in a few more X's here and there to make things look good. Then I said to myself, "Christ, has it come to *this*?"

If a popular magazine reports that married couples have sex 2.5 times per week, many couples feel they have to meet or exceed that statistic to feel "normal." The truth behind most surveys is that they represent an *average* of a wide range of ages and sexual frequencies varying from several times a day to several times a year. Each couple really has to work out for themselves the pace and pleasure of their sex lives. Infertility can upset this pace by speeding it up or slowing it down if the couple let it.

> From the beginning of our workup we were abstaining from intercourse for several days usually twice each month—once for tests and once to hit my ovulation time. We were "saving up sperm" to have tests and "saving up sperm" to try to make a baby. It became an incredibly precious body fluid to us. I used to think how awful it would be if after abstaining for 4 days my husband had a wet dream and all was lost!

It is a common occurrence for one or both partners of the couple to feel the desire for sex at times and to repress it because a "command performance" is only a few days off. As pointed out in chapter 4, there is no physiological rationale for "saving up sperm" more than 24 to 48 hours, which is the normal "recovery time" for a man to return to his usual sperm count. Frequency of relations seems to have a beneficial effect on motility, which is also very important to conception. If couples are blessed with sexual desire, they can do whatever they please until just before ovulation time; then an every-other-day regimen is suggested for 4 days. Once the temperature has risen (ovulation has occurred), they may return to the frequency they wish.

Impotence and Loss of Orgasm

Some men experience transient bouts of impotence in response to having to "perform," either for diagnostic tests or for sex at ovulation time. This can be extremely frightening and threatening to both partners. It may persist if the couple simply "try harder," as this is usually the cause in the first place. Probably the most common occurrence seen by doctors is inability to perform on the postcoital test (see pages 32 to 33). Many men also cannot masturbate on demand to produce a semen specimen in the doctor's office. The sensitive doctor will reschedule the postcoital test without comment and will allow men to produce their specimen at home. Bouts of impotence are far more common than most infertile couples realize, because it is hardly a subject they discuss lightly, even with a counselor or in a support group. When the problem *is* brought to light, it is very important for the doctor or counselor to take it as seriously as the couple does. The reassurance that such bouts are usually very temporary and short-lived is also important. Stress, anxiety, and depression can all take their toll on sexual performance. Help for the couple involves reducing these factors, taking some of the pressure off, a little vacation from the charts, tests, or attempts at treatment. The situation often corrects itself quickly.

It is as common for a woman to lose her libido and capacity for orgasm as it is for a man to have these problems. She is in a much different situation, however, as she is able to accept sex passively and to fake orgasm or simply admit it didn't happen. Neither loss of her desire or her orgasm will affect her ability to conceive. However, if she is honest with her partner, they can often help each other improve the quality of their relations, or at least can commiserate on the mutuality of their problem.

PROBLEMS AFTER FINAL DIAGNOSIS

If a final diagnosis of infertility is reached and one or both partners learn they have an incurable problem, it is understandable that a period of time may follow when feelings about sex are sad, negative, or threatening.

> I always felt that sex had other functions than procreation. I used birth control for years before my infertility was discovered. But at the back of my mind, when my husband and I made love, was the happy knowledge that someday, when the time and circumstances were right, this was the way we would create a baby. For a long time after the diagnosis we didn't feel like making love. In part, it was because of our general depression. In part, it was because of my new feelings of defectiveness. There was something so drastically wrong with my sexual equipment—how could anyone want to make love to me? But lurking behind it was also the feeling, "Why bother?" and "What for?"

Sex after infertility has been confirmed recalls many painful memories for each. The woman who has been thoroughly tested is reminded of each invasive procedure by the very position of standard intercourse. She may describe herself as feeling "hollow," "empty," and "numb" to feelings of pleasure. One woman who had a hysterectomy expressed her sadness for "all those sperm with no place to go." A man who found out he was sterile described the sex act as "shooting blanks." Infertile men have expressed their profound sadness over the cyclic ripening of eggs that will never be fertilized.

> After all we had been through, I just felt "burned out." Our sex life had been so hectic and frequent in the attempt to hit the right day that neither of us wanted any sex for a while. When he finally wanted to make love again, he was very gentle. I told him I just wasn't ready. I wasn't going to lie to him or "fake it." It took me a long time to get back to sex for its own sake. I wonder how many couples never get back.

Occasionally the reaction to a final diagnosis is just the opposite—overcompensation in the area of sex to oneself or one's partner that "at least we still have sex." Sometimes the need to prove sexuality strays outside the marriage.

> When I found the sperm count was so low that treatment was hopeless, I began seeing other women. I picked them up in bars, through my work, whatever I found. It felt good to have sex with anyone who didn't know about the problem. I even told one girl—who was afraid of getting pregnant—that I'd had a vasectomy! That felt really good.

> For several years after my hysterectomy I went through what I call my "Happy Hooker" phase. I felt like a eunuch inside, but by God, I still had a great bosom and I went all out to prove it—tight knit tops, deep-cut necklines—you can imagine for yourself. It sure turned the guys in the office on. All the women hated me. Then one day I caught a good look at myself in the washroom mirror and thought, "Here I am a happily married thirty-year-old looking like a common streetwalker." I decided it was time to clean up my act.

There is no easy cure for those who feel childbearing or impregnating are vital to sexuality. They generally realize after a time that self-deprecating actions are *not* helpful to either the marriage bond or to their own self-esteem. The person who is infertile must somehow come to understand and accept that sexuality is a *concept* he or she developed about being a man or a woman. If fertility was a key part of that concept, then the idea must be reworked. Fertility may be lost, but *sexuality cannot be lost*. A mother of ten and a mother of none have equal sexuality. The man with azoospermia and the man who fathers children into his eighties have equal sexuality. A nun and a priest have sexuality. *Sexuality may best be defined as the individual quality and character of being a woman or a man.* Sexuality is how a person *thinks* and *feels* about being the sex he or she is. A person has sexuality whether married or single, sexually active or celibate, fertile or infertile.

SEX FOR ITS OWN SAKE

Getting back to romantic, spontaneous, and pleasureful sex after infertility may take a long time. This subject has been the source of much discussion in both infertility counseling and RESOLVE support groups. Couples are very different in their approaches, varying from a "time heals all wounds" passivity to active pursuit of renewed orgasmic experience. Some general actions have been observed that seem to help the couple return to a mutually pleasureful sexual experience.

1. There is almost invariably a moratorium on sex after the final diagnosis, corresponding roughly to the period of grief, when both the man and the woman do not wish to have sexual relations. It helps if each respects the other's wishes about when they are ready to resume relations. If sexual tension builds in one partner before the other is ready to resume relations, masturbation alone or by the partner is often an acceptable outlet. Many couples find this a very tender time when they enjoy holding each other for comfort or exchanging massages for tactile pleasure.

2. Changing the location and time of sex can help. The bedroom can be declared off limits and so can the bedtime hour. The partners can use their imaginations to think up new times and places to have sex. This helps break the old and defeated pattern. It also restores some humor and spontaneity to the situation.

3. A change in the position of sexual relations can help. The worst position, because it evokes many negative feelings in the woman, is the "missionary position" of woman supine, man on top. Couples often experiment with new positions and variations on "outercourse," which include oral pleasuring or mutual masturbation. One advantage here is that ejaculation occurs outside the vagina, making connections with impregnation less likely. Many couples admit that they had once enjoyed these variations and had abandoned them because of the pursuit of pregnancy.

4. For the couple who feel unable to recover pleasureful sexual relations, or who never had them in the first place, marriage counseling or sexual therapy can often help. Because libido and potency are much more often mental than physical problems, talking about the feelings of infertility and marriage can uncover areas of conflict or unresolved issues and help the couple achieve a more intimate and pleasureful relationship.

5. The best help of all is believing in the *right* to have sex for its own sake! Religious training may hinder some people from this. Lingering feelings of guilt or unworthiness over infertility may inhibit others from this. It helps to have honest and open communications, with no faking or going along with something that isn't mutually satisfying. Good sex for its own sake is a gift, a way of communicating beyond words, a way of comforting and making each other feel loved.

SELF-IMAGE AND SELF-ESTEEM

Self-image (also called body image) is the concept people have about their bodies—both the visible exterior and the invisible interior. The person with a positive self-image feels attractive, normal, confident in his or her ability to perform physically or mentally, and acceptable to others. The person with a negative self-image feels just the opposite: unattractive, defective, unable to perform dependably either physically or mentally, and unacceptable to others. We develop our self-image very young and are fine-tuning it all our lives. A crisis such as infertility can trigger past issues of feelings about image as well as add new ones:

> When the doctor handed me the semen analysis results, which were disastrous, I had this incredible flashback to my earliest school days. *I was always the one chosen last for teams.* Here I was, not good enough for the team again.

One of the most common words used to describe self-image in infertility is *defective.* A defect exists. Something is not functioning as it should. The defect is invisible, carried inside. For the person with a negative self-image, the situation tends to confirm and compound the feeling that "my body can't do anything right." For the person with a very positive self-image, this may be the first time where his or her body has failed to perform, leading to great frustration. Self-image is often greatly helped by contact with other infertile people. One of the most common remarks heard at RESOLVE meetings is "Everyone here looks so *normal!*"

Self-esteem is an appropriate sense of pride and value in oneself. People with a healthy self-esteem are confident, optimistic, enjoy new situations and challenges, feel worthy of praise and acclaim that comes their way, and do not abuse themselves or allow others to hurt or abuse them. Poor self-esteem is characterized by feelings of lack of confidence, pessimism, inability to undertake risks or challenges, feeling unworthy or embarrassed in the face of praise, and a tendency toward self-abuse or allowing others to hurt and abuse them. This concept is also one developed in the early years of our lives. Like self-image, it is a formed concept that the person brings into the infertility situation and that may account for how he or she handles or fails to handle the crisis. People with healthy self-esteem tend to be rightfully upset and see the situation as something unfortunate that has happened to them. They often say, "But we *deserved* to have children!" People with poor self-esteem tend to accept infertility as proof of their unworthiness.

Part of the resolution of the crisis of infertility involves addressing the concepts of sexuality, self-image, and self-esteem and in some way understanding how they are linked with the infertility experience. The goal of successful resolution of infertility includes the ability to regain the feeling of being a fully functioning sexual person, adjustment of the self-image to incorporate the loss of fertility without feeling defective, and renewed self-esteem. Counseling and support groups can be a valuable tool in achieving these goals.

13. Special Concerns

The Moving Finger writes, and having writ,
Moves on; nor all your Piety nor Wit
Shall lure it back to cancel half a Line
Nor all your Tears wash out a Word of it.

RUBÁIYÁT OF OMAR KHAYYÁM

*T*here are many special areas within the subject of infertility that deserve detailed analysis. It is not possible to cover all these areas in depth, but five special concerns have been selected as representative in an attempt to give the reader increased insight and sensitivity and to portray the complexity of the situations that are lumped together under the term *infertility*. Indeed, they are as different from each other as night from day, and each carries its own unique pain and adjustments.

HYSTERECTOMY

Hysterectomy for the woman who has not been able to bear children or has not completed her family has great impact, both emotionally and physically. Almost without exception, doctors will strive to preserve the uterus and ovaries of a woman in her childbearing years, unless a problem so compromises the woman and her health that no choice is possible. Some examples of situations leading to hysterectomy in the young woman are cervical or uterine cancer; severe endometriosis, where the symptoms are intractable and

131

fertility is already presumed lost; infection that is rampant in the pelvic cavity and not responding to medical heroics; and massive hemorrhage, such as occasionally follows childbirth or miscarriage or ruptured ectopic pregnancy. Because such reasons for hysterectomy are extreme and sometimes sudden, the woman may not be able to address herself to the actual loss of her uterus (and often her ovaries) until she has recovered from what may have been a life-threatening situation. She may be told by those attempting to comfort her that she is lucky to have survived, and that is better off without the organ(s) that posed such a threat to her health. This may all be true, but it negates the feelings a woman must have over the loss of those organs, the loss of choices, and the loss of childbearing.

> I feel empty. It's like within me, where a uterus ought to be, there is a "black hole" of space. I feel mutilated and yet I am told I am lucky to be free of my pain at last. I do not feel lucky. I feel terribly, terribly depressed.

The uterus, though not necessary to life, is very symbolic. It symbolizes femininity and fertility. Even though it is internal and invisible, the uterus is not a silent organ like the liver or the spleen (for which most people feel little emotion). The uterus waxes and wanes with hormonal tides. Once a month it declares itself with a display of menstruation, accompanied by cramping and mood swings in some women. Many women state that they feel their sexual orgasm in "ripples or waves of sensation" in the uterus. Stimulation of the woman's nipples either in sex play or by a suckling infant is often accompanied by uterine contraction or waves of contractions that are, for many women, pleasureful. Therefore, the loss of the uterus has many meanings to the woman. She will not menstruate. She cannot conceive. She may feel differently about sexual relations and about foreplay. She may question the status of her womanhood. Certainly she has a right to acknowledge and grieve for these losses, whatever made them necessary.

> My own doctor was off and his associate came in. She was a woman in her forties. She seemed eager to cheer me up, I think, since I had been very depressed and weepy since my surgery. She said, "Just think! No more messy periods or buying tampons!" I started to cry and wanted to react—but felt defeated. How do you answer a statement as callous as that! . . . and from a *woman!*

Many young women review their hysterectomy for years to come and ask themselves the ultimate question: "Was it necessary?" In the overwhelming number of cases the answer is yes. For cases where there is doubt, or where outright mismanagement took place, the end result is nevertheless a fait accompli. This is one reason that a second opinion *before* surgery is extremely important if there is time. If opinions concur, the woman may undergo her surgery with a little more equanimity. If opinions differ, she may be spared unnecessary surgery. Women who have had the time to get second opinions seem to accept the surgery more readily. Unfortunately, the emergencies that often lead to early hysterectomy make second opinions difficult.

Feelings about a hysterectomy may surface at predictable times—at the anniversary of the event, upon the woman's being reminded of her friends who still menstruate, get pregnant, and give birth. One woman in a RESOLVE support group stated that there were two aisles of the supermarket she could not go down without crying—the "baby goods" aisle and the aisle with the sanitary napkins. Loss of the uterus in childbearing years is a special kind of infertility that carries a special kind of adjustment and grief. If a woman's ovaries have also been removed, she will have all of the feelings of the next category as well.

PREMATURE OVARIAN FAILURE

Loss of ovarian function by surgical, medical, or unknown causes before the natural cessation of their function at menopause is known as premature ovarian failure. It may occur in conjunction with a hysterectomy. Ovaries should not be routinely removed with a diseased uterus unless they are also diseased or there is a high risk of ovarian cancer in the woman's family. The argument that leaving good ovaries behind just provides another "potential cancer site" is not sound medicine. The benefit of the natural hormones and of a natural menopause to the woman far outweigh cancer risks unless the woman is of menopausal age. Sometimes the ovaries cease normal functioning for other reasons. Extensive surgery can impair ovaries and shorten their life span; repeated stimulation with powerful fertility drugs can blow them up or burn them out. Torsion of an ovary upon its blood supply can result in tissue death. In some women, the ovaries do not function properly from puberty. This is often characterized by very irregular cycles and scanty menstrual flow. This condition can be masked if birth control pills are prescribed early and a woman takes them for a long time.

> For years I suspected there might be something wrong with me. I menstruated very, very rarely. But when I asked doctors about it, they told me not to worry: that it was a common problem; that it probably meant nothing; that, besides, tests were expensive and time-consuming and pointless until I actually wanted to become pregnant. In the meantime they cavalierly prescribed hormones to "trigger" menstruation and the Pill for birth control. I know that it is very

unlikely that my premature ovarian failure was caused by anything they did or didn't do. I know too that—even if a doctor had told me when I was sixteen that my fertile years were not likely to last long—I would certainly not have chosen to have a child then! But still I am angry at the way they brushed off my concern, at the readiness with which they prescribed drugs, at their automatic recommendation of the Pill when I sought birth control.

One of the very unfortunate associations with premature ovarian failure is the word *menopause*. Menopause is more than a medical word referring to the cessation of menstruation. It has become a sociological word that evokes negative images of women suffering "hot flashes," experiencing depressions, drying up in their sexual functions, and becoming *old*. The fact that this image is not true for the great majority of women in their menopause does not diminish the strength of the stereotype.

Two years ago, when I was twenty-three, a doctor told me I was menopausal. "I hate to hit you between the eyes with this," he began, "but . . ." The word *menopause* no longer causes me pain. Since that day in his office I've learned to separate its meaning as a medical term from all the stereotyped images it conjures up. But I've also learned that there's another, less loaded term to describe my medical situation, premature ovarian failure—and I wish the doctor had shown the sensitivity to use it instead. I walked into his office at twenty-three, with my childbearing years all ahead of me. I left at fifty half an hour later, my fertile years somehow gone without a trace. Looking at my wedding picture, I still sometimes think, "How young I looked then!" Looking in the mirror, I still have to remind myself that I am only twenty-five.

The medical term for removal of either the testes in men or the ovaries in women is *castration*. Ovaries are symbolic of femininity and fertility just as the uterus is, but they are more silent and unfelt. Most women focus their grief on the loss of fertility first. The loss of femininity, real or imagined, is more difficult to communicate. Most doctors will start a young woman immediately on a form of *estrogen replacement therapy* (ERT) and assurances are given that she will feel "as good as ever." While this is generally the case, the adjustment from having natural body hormones to taking estrogen by mouth is a daily reminder that this is a most "unnatural" situation.

I take a form of the birth control pill to supply the estrogens my body no longer makes. I have to keep them out on my bathroom counter to remember to take them (if I forget even one day I get a miniperiod). I am divorced and dating now, and more than one man has remarked, "Oh, you're on the Pill!" And I just say yes. One time I happened to have my pill pack in my purse when I was on vacation and as I reached for my checkbook it fell out on the counter in front of half a dozen people. I felt so mortified—then sort of "proud" as I realized these people, if they noticed at all, were not seeing my *ovaries* fall out of my purse. They would have assumed I was fertile and sexually active!

Premature loss of ovarian function can lead to uncomfortable and possibly dangerous problems in the young woman. Most common symptoms are "hot flashes"—waves of flushing and warmth often accompanied by sweating. These are caused indirectly by the high FSH level of the body, as the pituitary sends its signal to the ovary, which cannot respond, and the pituitary sends a much stronger FSH signal. Other troublesome symptoms are vaginal dryness and eventual atrophy, insomnia, nervous irritability, and depression. Perhaps more significantly, but on a more gradual basis, calcium will be lost from the bones, a condition that may lead to *osteoporosis*.

The debate over estrogen replacement therapy rages on in medical circles. One week a medical journal carries a study proving that ERT is conducive to certain cancers; then the next issue features a study proving that ERT is *protective* against those very cancers. Most hotly debated are cancers of the uterus and breast. Doctors seem to agree that the young woman who has lost her ovarian function should have estrogen replacement at least until the time of her natural menopause. In the young woman, the benefits of ERT are control of hot flashes, reduction of vaginal dryness or atrophy, and avoidance of osteoporosis. If a woman has her uterus, the conservative management is the minimum dosage of an estrogen/progestin combination that will keep her symptom-free, given in a cycle with one week off for shedding of the uterine lining or menstruation. This seems to reduce the hazard of uterine cancer. There is no current evidence that ERT increases risk of breast cancer. ERT may also be protective in retarding the aging process of the cardiovascular system in the young woman. This "protection" appears to reverse to a risk if ERT is continued past the age of normal menopause, and it dramatically presents a risk for women who smoke.

Women who prefer not to take estrogen after ovarian failure report some control over symptoms by taking extra calcium in their diet, exercising regularly, and controlling their weight. Also, there appears to be truth to the "use it or lose it" adage in that regular sexual relations tend to prevent vaginal dryness and atrophy. The body adjusts to loss of ovarian function over time and most symptoms subside.

SECONDARY INFERTILITY

Technically called *secondary infertility*, the inability to conceive again after one or more successful pregnancies is a distressing experience. It can occur after any number of successful pregnancies, but the couples who are most often distraught are those who have one child and wish to have another.

If you think there is pressure to have your first child, you ought to see the kind of pressure there is to have your *second*. An only child is seen by many as worse than no child at all. And since you conceived once, people are convinced you will be able to conceive again. The grace period for us was about three years. After that people started making remarks like "Isn't it about time to have another?"

Society has certain expectations of the adult couple. They are expected to bear *children*. A single child is not enough. Perhaps this conviction has its roots in the days when families had to be very big so that some would survive the disease, malnutrition, and dangers of life. Infant mortality still approaches 50 percent in some countries of the world. A single child poses a great threat to family continuity.

Couples who have conceived once with relative ease are naturally baffled when the same does not hold true the second time around. The reasons for secondary infertility may be any of those for primary infertility and are presumed to have developed or worsened in the interval between the first and second effort. A very common emotion in secondary infertility is *frustration*. The couple "controlled" reproduction once but now it eludes them. There may also be guilt or anger, especially if birth control was practiced or an abortion occurred in the interval. Secondary infertility is cured at the same rate as primary infertility, in about half of all cases. Therefore active investigation of the problem with a qualified specialist is recommended. However, for some the verdict will be negative, and they must face the prospect of raising a single child or looking into an alternative such as adoption.

One of the most poignant pressures in secondary infertility comes from the single children themselves. From the time they realize that their other friends have siblings and that other parents have pregnancies, children may beg, wheedle, and plead for a little brother or sister. As they are often too young to understand even the mechanisms of *normal* reproduction, little children cannot grasp the concept of infertility or the reason why "we can't make any more babies." They may interpret this as "we *will* not make any more babies," which may cause their redoubled efforts at begging. It may make them secretly wonder if it was because they were so difficult or bad that Mommy and Daddy cannot face the thought of a second child.

The worst and most painful pressure we faced came from our daughter, Annette. She is a thoughtful and sensitive child and at six years of age now loves to "mother" all the little toddlers on the block. I found her crying in her bed one night because she wants a baby brother so much. I explained for the millionth time that I would love one too, but that my body could not make a baby anymore. She cried many times over this, and I often cried with her as I comforted her. She was not blaming us, or angry—which I would have found easier to bear. She was just so very sad and lonely.

Many couples with secondary infertility express great fear that something will happen to the child they have. *Overprotection* can result, with negative effects on both the child and the parents. They may also push their child to be a high achiever, since all their hopes rest on the accomplishments of one child. These actions stem from very understandable feelings. Naturally each illness, accident, or threat to their child will trigger protective feelings. Each milestone will be met by a combination of pride, fear, and nostalgia.

I sit and look at her and think, "She is *irreplaceable*." In a sense each child is one of a kind and irreplaceable. But when fertility is gone and one is all you've got, that fact is so absolute. Now I worry over her crossing two streets on her way to kindergarten. How will it be when she has her first date, learns to drive, goes away to college? Each milestone rings so final. *We will never go this way again.*

Couples with a single child because of infertility are being joined in increasing numbers by couples who have a single child by choice. The "only child" is no longer a social phenomenon that sets teachers, neighbors, and relatives to whispering. As with other social changes—more children of divorce, more children whose mothers work, and so on—stereotypes break down when numbers increase. The single child may one day be commonplace. This is small comfort to the couple who wished to have more, but it may ease their child's adjustment to the situation.

THE "NORMAL INFERTILE" COUPLE

For approximately 10 percent of couples with infertility, no physical or metabolic reason is ever found to account for the fact that they do not conceive despite years of effort. These patients are among the most challenging and baffling an infertility specialist encounters. They are among the most deserving of sympathy and support, as their emotional, physical, and financial expenditure toward achieving pregnancy is never-ending. These patients have been labeled as "normal infertile" by doctors, though, in the words of one well-known Boston specialist, "The so-called normal infertile couple obviously is not normal or they would not have an infertility problem."*

* Robert Kistner, M.D., "The Infertile Woman," *American Journal of Nursing* (November 1973): 1937.

Is It Psychological?

Because there is no definite physical finding—no hopelessly blocked tubes or zero sperm count—the normal infertile couple may fall prey to suggestions that the problem is psychological. This suggestion is cruel beyond words. The visible signs of anxiety, depression, and frustration from an unceasing battle are mistaken as the *cause* instead of the *effect* of the problem. When the suggestion originates from family or friends, it is presumably based in part on a sincere desire to help, and in part on that old superstition that in order to conceive a couple must *relax!* "Take a second honeymoon," encourages Mother, knowingly. "Quit your job," says Aunt Fanny to the wife. Or if the wife is fretting at home unemployed, "Why don't you go to work?" The clergyman suggests, "Put the problem in the Lord's hands." The family doctors suggests a tipple of sherry before bedtime. All are cunning folklore ways of encouraging the couple to . . . *RELAX!!!*

The suggestion that infertility may be *psychogenic* (caused by the mind) may come from professional quarters as well. Some doctors are unable to accept that the science of infertility is not yet perfect. If they cannot find a problem to treat, they may imply to the patient that "stress" might be the problem. Psychiatrists and therapists of the Freudian school may interpret infertility as a subconscious wish to avoid pregnancy or parenting. Adoption workers point to the fact that some people become pregnant after adopting— proof that they were more relaxed. The truth is that there is the same pregnancy rate for infertile couples who adopt as those who do not. There is a 5 percent spontaneous cure rate (pregnancy without any treatment) at play in all but absolute infertility cases. This 5 percent is behind the stories of "miracle babies" conceived when all hope was lost.

It is probably true that being relaxed and carefree has a beneficial effect on health in general—maybe even on infertility. But it is also true that women conceive under the most stressful of circumstances: during rape, during famine and starvation, in severe psychotic states, and in the presence of abhorrence of sex and/or the sexual partner. People who really wish to help the normal infertile couple should realize that blaming the victim is counterproductive. It will drive the anxiety and stress only higher and will add guilt, if the couple truly believe they are doing something to make themselves infertile.

What seems to help the normal infertile couple most is a safe and nonjudgmental place to share their feelings of despair and frustration. Support groups work very well for some, although they are at risk at being exposed to people who are getting concrete diagnoses and having success with treatments. They often feel "stuck" as they see even their infertile friends move on to new levels. Individual or couple therapy may feel safer, and it allows the couple to focus completely on their own particular pain.

When to Say Enough!

It is this author's experience that infertile couples do not search for a pregnancy as much as they search for an *answer*. Human beings have a heartening stamina to stand up to stress and pain, if only they can ultimately know the reason for it.

> The big problem with normal infertility is making the decision to stop trying. I knew we could continue going to doctors for years. I can't continue to live this way. It is necessary at some point to say, "The hell with it!"

When an answer to infertility is found, and is absolute, most couples have a courageous capacity to experience their loss, to grieve over it, and then to get on with the business of living. If a reason is found that can be treated, as in half of the cases, the couple will experience their longed-for pregnancy and birth. In both these situations, the outcome is eventually definite. In the case of the normal infertile couple, there is nothing conclusive. Years can be spent in a wasteland of suspended animation. There is no pregnancy. There is no known loss, so they cannot grieve and move on. They may shop from doctor to doctor, even country to country, in search of their answer.

It is not easy to abandon the search without an answer. Nor is it easy to turn to an alternative, such as adoption. There is still too much energy caught up in the hope for pregnancy. One event that ends the search and precipitates grief is menopause. It is logical that women (and couples) who have never truly given up hope will experience menopause intensely. The couple who have delayed this long in looking into adoption may find agency doors shut to people their age. Even in midlife and beyond, couples may be troubled by depression over the children they never had and the answer that never came.

Some couples find they cannot live with the monthly tension of wondering if the woman will get pregnant, and they take active control over their situation.

> I got so preoccupied with my infertility that everything suffered—my job, my friendships, especially my marriage. I finally asked my doctor for a diaphragm. After six months of using it and being released from the constant anxiety of infertility, I found my whole outlook had vastly improved. I have gone off birth control again, feeling I can cope for a while again. But I plan to use it whenever I get upset. It is the only way I know of controlling the anxiety. If I am not pregnant by the age of thirty-five, I will seriously consider having a tubal ligation to end this worry forever.

> We would be hypocrites to talk about being childfree and be secretly plotting my temperature graph every day. Once we decided to take control over our fertility situation, we felt great relief. We use birth control now. The best thing was

rediscovering sex for its own sake. Eventually one of us will have a sterilization, ironic as that sounds. It is the only way we can honestly espouse a childfree life and get on with our careers.

The normal infertile couple have exaggerated emotional needs caused by the perpetual cycles of hope and despair they endure. They are particularly vulnerable to exploitation by fads, quackery, and claims of some of the new technologies. Some nontraditional cures they may explore include megavitamin therapy, acupuncture, herbalists, hypnosis, astrology, faith healers, special diets, and meditation. Most of these are benign and do no physical harm, even if they do no good. But no claims have yet been substantiated that any of these means will result in pregnancy. It is interesting to note that both in vitro fertilization and gamete interfallopian transfer programs have been most successful in treating this population.

ATTEMPTING PREGNANCY AFTER THIRTY-FIVE

Current statistics reveal that more and more couples are waiting until the years after the age of thirty-five to begin having their families. Women are taking the time to complete their educations, work at a career for a number of years, and establish a financial and emotional base upon which to build a family. Couples find a two-salary income no longer a luxury, but a necessity if they wish to buy a house, travel, and have some material comforts. The couple also have a chance to test their relationship for a number of years before attempting to bring children into the picture. Few would argue that delaying marriage and childbearing both have distinct advantages from a financial and emotional point of view. The problem is that biologically a woman is maximally fertile in her mid-twenties, and that there are significant risks and problems in waiting until the age of thirty-five or later to begin testing fertility.

A woman has an increased chance of infertility for every year after the age of thirty she delays childbearing. Endometriosis is known to progress and become more of a problem in older women; there is a higher incidence of fibroid tumors of the uterus; if there have been multiple sexual relationships before marriage, there is an increased risk of sexually transmitted disease and pelvic disease. Women past thirty often have a less regular pattern of ovulation and may have diminished quality of ova. If a woman does conceive later in life, she has a higher risk of giving birth to a child with Down's syndrome or other birth defects. It used to be assumed that maternal age alone was responsible for increased risk of Down's syndrome. It is now known that an older father may also be responsible. The risk of a man producing an offspring with Down's syndrome doubles after age fifty-five. *

The couple who do not readily conceive after the age of thirty-five have less time to engage in a proper investigation and attempted treatment of their case. The "biological clock" is ticking loudly in the background as they begin the search for the problem. Even the most aggressive approach to investigation may take months to complete; attempts at certain therapies, because they involve monthly cycles, can take over a year to have a sufficient trial. All the while, if the couples are not also pursuing adoption alternatives, they are rapidly becoming too old to be considered for an infant adoption by many agency's standards.

The question of what to do about a possible defective fetus should be addressed by the older couple before the woman becomes pregnant. If they are unable to face an abortion, then there is no point to having an amniocentesis to detect Down's syndrome (and a number of other birth defects). If they feel unable to cope with raising a retarded or defective child, then perhaps they should choose adoption over pregnancy.

Amniocentesis can be done only between the fourteenth and eighteenth weeks of pregnancy. It is a safe procedure and accurate when performed by a skilled doctor. The risk of spontaneous abortion or damage to the fetus is only about .05 percent. Ultrasound is used to locate the fetus within the amniotic sac. A thin needle is inserted through the abdomen into the uterus. (The procedure is usually painless, although it may cause slight uterine contractions.) The needle is then guided into the amniotic sac around the baby, using ultrasound. About one ounce of fluid is withdrawn for inspection. This fluid contains cells from the fetus and therefore can show the fetus's genetic makeup. It takes about three to five weeks for the cells to grow in a culture to the point where they can be examined for chromosomes. A normal test will show 46 matched chromosomes in each cell. Down's syndrome will show that chromosome 21 has three strands of DNA instead of two. Amniocentesis is accurate about 90 percent of the time. There are more than 100 other tests that can be run on the fluid drawn during amniocentesis. Unfortunately, there are another 700 birth defects that cannot be identified in this way. However, Down's syndrome is by far the most common, comprising 70 to 80 percent of spontaneous birth defects. If a woman chooses to abort her pregnancy based on an abnormal testing result, she is already well into her second trimester and the procedure will have to be done by a chemical induction, carried out in the hospital. While there is a minimal risk to her health or future fertility, it is a difficult event to undergo, and people will be

* Joseph H. Bellina, M.D., and Josleen Wilson, *You Can Have a Baby* (New York: Crown Publishers, 1985), p. 335.

aware of the pregnancy and the loss of it. What the couple choose to tell others is a personal decision requiring careful thought.

> I was thirty-seven when we finally conceived our first baby. We were in agreement about having an amniocentesis and so I felt it wise not to tell anyone I was pregnant until we were "sure" the baby was all right. This was very sad, in a way, after all the time we had wanted a baby. From the fourth month on it became increasingly hard to conceal my growing abdomen. I was feeling the baby kick and move. We were trying so hard to be detached so we wouldn't have to grieve if an abortion was necessary. The hardest weeks were from the test to the results. I was then very aware of my baby; only the most artful dressing kept my figure concealed. When the test was normal we immediately told everyone. But I felt cheated out of four months of "expectancy" and it took some time to begin letting myself feel a bond to my baby. If I had it to do over again, I would tell people right away and would deal with an abortion as if it were a miscarriage, if it had to happen.

There is a new technique for fetal testing that samples chorionic villi instead of amniotic fluid. A small sample of the placenta is taken through the cervix and can be examined as early as 8 weeks of gestation, and an early answer may be obtained within one week. The risk appears no greater than that of amniocentesis in the hands of an expert. It is not yet widely available beyond major medical centers.

Reduced fertility and risk of birth defects are only two of the problems facing the woman over thirty-five. Her own health and ability to carry a pregnancy to term are in greater jeopardy than in the younger woman. She is more at risk for pre-eclampsia than the thirty-year-old woman. Pregnancy may be beset with problems, aches, and pains, not seen as frequently in younger women.

> Each day of my pregnancy I was plagued with nausea. There were worse times, like the first and last 6 weeks, but never a day better than a constant vomitous feeling in my stomach. Yet I did not feel I had the privilege of complaining. I had even said a number of times that I'd gladly be sick every day of a pregnancy just to have a baby! I was miserable. The only thing that seemed to help, ironically, was eating to relieve the churnings and to fight the fears I had. Sixty pounds attest to their magnitude.

Labor is considerably longer in the older woman having her first baby. Cesarean sections are much more common in older women. The woman over thirty is more at risk for stillbirth, placental problems, fibroids of the uterus, and fetal distress. All can result in the decision to do a cesarean. Most older women are considered to be carrying a "premium" baby—perhaps one of a kind, and the doctor will choose the delivery method that gives the highest probability of a healthy baby.

The older couple having a "miracle baby" often feel they have no right to complain about pregnancy, delivery, the postpartum recovery, or parenting in general. After all, this is their dream come true. How could they possibly complain! Fears about parenting begin the moment the baby is handed to his or her parents. This very small, reddened, wrinkled, puffy-eyed, pointy-headed person may seem very little payoff after years of infertility investigation and treatment. Love does not spring automatically from their hearts at the first touch. The bonding process is a gradual one, and some feel it takes more time if parents have romanticized and idealized the moment of birth for many years. *Postpartum depression* is seen in a number of women who have had extensive infertility experiences. After all, no single event or infant can instantly make up for years of longing and tribulation. In actual fact, an infant is not going to make up for anything, or *give* anything to parents for many months. He or she is going to make demands on them and not consider their feelings or needs in the slightest!

Parents of a "miracle baby" often feel they have to perform to a higher standard of parenting than other people do. They have to do everything just right. They are reluctant to leave the child with a sitter or in day care if the mother returns to work. Their need or desire to return to work is hard to reconcile with the years they longed for a baby in their home. The result is *guilt*. If this child is the only one the woman will ever conceive, they share many of the feelings of the secondary infertility situation, including a tendency to overprotect their child and pressure it into being all things to them. In a sense, both the parents and the child conceived under these circumstances are "set up" for unrealistic expectations in life.

14. Alternatives for the Infertile Couple

Flow, flow, flow,
the current of life is ever onward.

KOBODAISHI

*T*here are four basic alternatives to remaining childless, and none of them is an easy decision to make. *Adoption,* the traditional alternative route to family building is harder now than ever before, especially if a healthy young infant is desired. *Donor insemination* is gaining in popularity and acceptance for those couples with a male factor problem, and *surrogate motherhood* if there is a female factor problem, but these require special adjustments that not all couples can make. The fourth alternative, *childfree living,* is also gaining in popularity and is a viable choice for many couples. Each of these areas will be examined in depth.

ADOPTION

Until the 1970s, adoption of a healthy infant of one's own race was a reliable and relatively easy alternative to being involuntarily childless. The situation has changed with the increasing availability of birth control, the availability of legal abortion, and most of all because over 70 percent of single women who choose to bear their babies are now keeping them. Babies and children available for adoption vary greatly from one part of the country to another and from rural to urban areas. Couples who are assertive and well informed can still find and adopt local babies, but the waiting lists in traditional agency adoption may now be more than 5 years long. This poses problems for couples who wish to have children while they are still young enough to enjoy them, as the infertility may have been discovered in the years after thirty, and attempts at treatment may have eaten up more years. Getting a second child by this route is sometimes out of the question, either because agencies have a "one to a customer" approach, or because the couple have passed the age of forty, when many agencies will no longer place an infant in their home.

Many couples have turned to other than traditional agency adoptions in an effort to speed up the placement and fulfill their parenting desires. Some other types of babies and children available for adoption are:

1. International infants and children
2. Special-needs children (older, siblings, handicapped)
3. Legal-risk adoptions
4. Private or identified adoptions

Each of these categories has its advocates and its pros and cons, and each will be discussed in detail.

Traditional Agency Adoption

The couple who turn to adoption as an alternative have usually explored their infertility to a nontreatable conclusion. It is hoped that they have dealt with their normal feelings of anger, guilt, and grief over this obstacle and have concluded that *parenthood*, not just pregnancy, is their primary goal. The couple are often not in concert in exploring alternatives. One may be eager while the other is reluctant. Confidence is often gained by "information gathering" on the types of adoption and adoptable babies and children available. Almost all couples begin by calling a local adoption agency to learn what the situation is.

Most good adoption agencies offer informational meetings to those who inquire. These may be held once a month or less often, but they give a couple a chance to ask questions and learn about adoption before they ever enter into the process. Those who are still interested at the end of a meeting may be allowed to fill out a preliminary application form, which puts them on a waiting list—or in some cases, a wait for the waiting list. The fact that the waiting list may be five to six years long does not deter most couples, although it sends them searching to other agencies and other types of adoption for additional information. Most waiting lists are very inflated by couples who are on every waiting list that would take them. This practice is encouraged by parent advocates, since as soon as an agency begins to consider them seriously and conduct a "home study" at that point the couple must take their names off other lists. It does, however, mean that the agency that places 25 babies a year and has a waiting list of 200 people will not necessarily be an eight-year wait!

A couple may contact the agency from time to time to see how they are progressing on the waiting list and to reinforce their eagerness. When they come to a point where a placement might be likely within a finite time frame—six to twelve months—they will be asked to come in for a home study. This innocuous phrase often strikes terror in the hearts of infertile couples. They feel as if they must pass muster, prove themselves in order to be awarded a baby. It is a time fraught with emotions and irrational fears even when the adoption worker is nonthreatening and helpful. The purpose of the home study is to determine if the couple can provide a safe and nurturing environment for the baby they seek. Questions will be asked about their infertility, their feelings about their infertility, their individual motivations for adopting, and the state of their marriage. Often questions are asked about each partner's childhood and feelings about *their* parents. At some point the adoption worker will come to see them in their house, not to "inspect" the premises, but to see the environment and life-style their home reflects. A home study may be over in a matter of several sessions or it may go on extensively. Sometimes the initial meetings are done with a group of couples together. After the home study, the couples are presented on paper for approval by the agency. Approval is usually assured to couples who complete the home study. Those with serious conflicts or problems will be offered counseling along the way. Some couples "select themselves out," realizing adoption is not right for them.

Once the couple are approved, the agency goes to work searching for the type of baby the couple have indicated they want. It helps if the couple have not been too restrictive on sex, age of baby, and background (such as college-educated parents). Some couples are able to be flexible on minor health problems or a child of an ethnic origin other than their own. Some couples will consider a child of another race, or a multiracial one. Whatever the wishes of the couple, the agency will then set to work searching its caseload of pregnant mothers or foster homes for an appropriate child.

The couple will receive a call when a baby is found for them. They are often invited in to see the baby within a day or two, and if everything goes well, they take the child home. Adoption workers will continue to monitor the placement with home visits for the next few months. In most states a couple can go to court and legally adopt the baby within six months of placement. The child is then legally theirs.

Costs of traditional agency adoptions are from $3,000 to $6,000 in most cases. This fee pays the agency overhead, the adoption worker's time, legal fees, and sometimes subsidizes foster home or pregnant-mother expenses. In *no* state is it legal to sell a baby or child.

International Adoption

Some couples cannot cope with a five-year wait and feel they can happily parent a child of a different race or culture. Another variable in international adoption is that there may be little or no prenatal care and little information about the background of the birth-parents. Some countries that are currently supplying orphaned and abandoned babies for adoption are Korea, Colombia, Peru, El Salvador, Chile, and India. Southeast Asia was a source of many adoptable babies during the Vietnam War and some children still come from this area. The situation changes dramatically from year to year. Countries close down, others open their doors.

In order to adopt a child from another country, a couple must have an approved home study by a local agency and must supply considerable paperwork to the liaison in the country of adoption. The fee is higher, often $6,000 to $10,000. Sometimes the couple are required to travel to the country to pick up the child. In other cases the children come with "escorts."

A couple that have been approved will usually learn of a baby or child in the country available to them. They may be sent a photo and small "brief" on the child. They accept the child (or not) based on this information. There are frequently concerns about health, nutritional status, parasites, and conditions in the orphanage or foster site. Couples should have worked out their feelings about adopting a baby that will not resemble them, and that may wish to identify with his or her birth culture and race in the future. Meeting with local support groups of parents who have adopted internationally can be very reassuring. The resources organization and section at the end of this book gives the names of organizations that can help couples get in touch with others who have adopted internationally.

Special-Needs Children

It is ironic that, while healthy infants and toddlers are in very short supply, there are others who must actually wait for a home and family to call their own. Children of "special needs" of all races exist in every state. Some types of children that fall into this category include children over the age of six, sibling groups needing to be placed together, children with serious medical handicaps, children with mental retardation, children with emotional disturbances, and those with learning disabilities. The right of these children to a permanent, loving home is beyond question, but it is a difficult first-parenting experience for most childless couples to consider. It requires great confidence and flexibility to adopt a first child from this category. Add to this that the failure rate for special-needs placements is almost 50 percent in most states, even with the best matching and counseling. Such a failure, known by the euphemism "a disruption" in adoption, is devastating to both would-be parents and child. Many agencies prefer experienced parents for these children, but they are not to be ruled out by the couple who are researching every opportunity in adoption. These adoptions often cost very little, as they are subsidized by the state, and often medical or counseling expenses are subsidized as well.

Legal-Risk Adoption

Most legal-risk babies and children are prime adoptable candidates with the exception that they are not yet legally free for adoption. When the expectation is that the birth-parent(s) will surrender rights on a child, he or she may be placed temporarily as a foster child with a couple until they can proceed with adoption. Many of these children come from troubled homes, and in some cases there may be neglect or abuse involved. As the name implies, there is legal risk that the surrender for adoption will be delayed, or may never be forthcoming, but in the great majority of these cases, the couple go on to a happy adoption. Such placements are not for the fainthearted, and all aspects of the case must be fully disclosed. The cost of this kind of adoption is usually subsidized, as in special needs, and the waiting period may be brief. The agencies will still need an approved home study. For those couples who wish to speed up the adoption process and are willing to take risks, this type of adoption may be an answer. Couples should ask about this type at any traditional agency, as most have legal-risk babies from time to time.

Private Adoption

More and more birth-mothers are choosing not to deal with adoption agencies but to deal directly with infertile couples by means of an intermediary— usually a lawyer or doctor. Infertile couples are doing the same thing, sometimes advertising their need for a baby in local magazines or newspaper classifieds, or doing mass mailings to doctors and laywers in their area. Private adoption, also called independent adoption, is legal in all but 6 states. Because no formal home study is done in most cases, traditional adoption advocates feel the interests of the child may not be protected in this type of adoption. Couples who choose it often feel agencies are too slow and arbitrary and decide to "go it alone." Birth-mothers often choose this route because they feel they have more control over the kind of home their baby is placed in, and they may, in fact, insist on meeting and screening the applicants.

There are several pitfalls for all parties to be concerned about in private adoption. First, if anonymity between birth-parents and adoptive parents is important, the intermediary must be scrupulously careful to preserve this. If it is waived, the danger exists of ongoing visits and communications between the birth-parent(s) and child. Some adoptive parents are comfortable with this; others are not. Second, private adoptions tend to cost more than traditional adoptions. Since it is illegal to "sell a baby," the infertile couple is ostensibly paying for the mother's medical care and the intermediary fee. Both should be set at the outset so the couple know what they are getting into financially. The costs can be as high as $15,000 or more. Finally, as with surrogate motherhood, there is a real risk that the birth-parent will renege on her surrender of the baby and leave the infertile couple with nothing but heartbreak.

In states where private adoption is illegal, a variation called "identified adoption" has sprung up. A couple still locate a birth-mother who wishes to give up a baby, on their own, with or without an intermediary. Then they call an agency and ask to be home studied for *this particular baby.* They will generally go to the head of the list, since agencies have so few babies to place. If the home study is successful, the adoption then proceeds as if it were a traditional adoption. This negates the agency claim that private adoption doesn't serve the best interest of the child because there is no home study. Not all agencies will do identified adoption, but more are realizing that it is a viable alternative to their woefully long waiting lists and small supply of babies.

Black-Market Adoption

Sometimes what looks like a legitimate adoption situation turns into nothing more than "baby selling" for the profit of a birth-parent, an intermediary, or both. Sometimes infertile couples are so desperate in their quest for a baby that they knowledgeably enter into the black market. The first clue that a baby is a black-market product is the extremely high expense. Fees in excess of $25,000 are not uncommon. The second tip-off is the frequent anonymity of the intermediary, who may operate out of a post office box and use a fictitious name. The intermediary will often demand a large amount of money "up front" and will initiate all calls so as not to be traced. Couples have been exploited out of huge sums and have failed to receive a baby. Some couples have received a baby, only to be plagued by repeated blackmail threats by the birth-mother or the intermediary. Some babies placed in black-market operations have actually been kidnapped for sale. Needless to say, black-market adoption is not only illegal, it is dangerous.

* * *

It is important for couples considering adoption to become as well informed as possible about all their options. The list of readings and resources at the end of this book offers an excellent start. Couples must realize that adoption is not an answer for everyone. It does not remove the fact of one's infertility. It does not give a couple a child with their genetic heritage. It does not, obviously, provide a pregnancy experience, nor in many cases, an early infant experience. If adopting a baby is going to feel "second best" to the couple, this cannot fail to be communicated to the child over the years and is an unfair and unhealthy situation for all.

> Adoption eased the pain of childlessness, but one fact is irrevocable. I will never be able to experience a pregnancy. I will never be able to reproduce those genes I find so adorable in my husband. Adoption does not cure infertility.

On the other hand, adoption does allow a couple to have the rewarding and challenging experience of parenting. The children who come into the welcoming arms of adoptive parents are as dissimilar in health, race, and ethnic background as can be. Some families have children of several different cultural backgrounds, or with several kinds of special needs. Often as a couple gain experience, they feel more open to challenges beyond the healthy local infant. When adoption works, the parents grow to love their children as intensely as they ever could have loved a baby born to them. There is often a mystical kind of fatalism that this *particular* child was meant to be theirs, because both were in need at the same point in time and miraculously found each other.

> They talk of the miracle of birth. Yes, birth is a miracle. I will tell you another kind of miracle. A child was born in Can Tho province of Vietnam and abandoned at birth. He was found and cared for by the devoted nurses and sisters first in an orphanage there, and later in Saigon. He was declared eligible for adoption at three months when he looked stable enough in health that they thought he might live. Twelve thousand miles away, in Boston, we applied to our local adoption agency and also to an agency in Colorado that dealt with Vietnamese orphans. After waiting what seemed to be an eternity, we were called one night about this little black Vietnamese boy. Without hesitation, without a picture, on blind instinct and faith we said yes! Two months later we received him into our arms at Kennedy Airport in New York City. *That is also a miracle.*

ARTIFICIAL INSEMINATION BY DONOR

Artificial insemination by donor (AID) is not a new procedure. It has been practiced in animal husbandry for many years, with the earliest accounts of insemination in animals dating back to Arabian sources in the fourteenth century. It was not until 1890, in the greatest secrecy, that artificial insemination by donor in humans was performed, although one must suspect that donor insemination by discreet adultery has been practiced by women from earliest history. Since the first accounts of successful donor insemination, the procedure has gained acceptance and the medical-legal controls it requires, until today it is estimated that as many as 15,000 babies may be conceived by this procedure in America annually. Since records are kept confidential, it is impossible to verify this statistic, which may actually be higher.

Moral, Ethical, and Religious Concerns

Artificial insemination by donor (AID) is not morally, ethically, or religiously acceptable to all couples, or to their doctors. The Roman Catholic church and Orthodox Judaism both forbid its use, though in the latter case the offspring is seen as legitimate, while in Roman Catholicism, the offspring is seen as illegitimate and the act itself as adultery. Reform Judaism and major Protestant religions have taken a neutral stand on AID, feeling it is up to the individual conscience of the participants to decide what is right for themselves.

Legally, AID is still in limbo. To date, only a handful of states have statutes specifically governing artificial insemination. All these statutes more or less agree that successful AID, performed by a licensed physician, with written consent of both members of the couple, results in a legitimate child. Even if the couple subsequently divorce, the child born of AID will receive child support, if necessary, in those states. In other states, laws either do not exist or are unclear.

AID is an alternative to be considered when the male has an infertility problem that proves untreatable, and the female appears to be fertile. Sometimes the situation is a genetic disorder that the male partner is apt to pass along to offspring. Couples may choose AID over adoption because waiting lists are very long, because they wish to share the pregnancy and birth experience together, and because they will know at least half the child's genetic heritage and be able to provide an ideal prenatal environment. While the technique of donor insemination is very simple, the decision to have a child by this route is very complex. Often a couple need counseling and much reassurance to come to a point of readiness. In some cases, couples will decide it is *not* a viable alternative and will turn to another way of having a family. It is important that the doctor and staff of facilities that provide AID be sensitive to the difficulty of this decision and respect the couples' need to take their time and make their own choice.

The Technique of Donor Insemination

The couple considering AID generally come to a clinic and discuss the procedure with the doctor and possibly a counselor. Questions a couple will want to ask include:

1. Who are donors?
2. How are donors screened for genetic history and current infections?
3. Is fresh or frozen semen used?
4. What is the expected cost per cycle?
5. How many inseminations per month are done?
6. Is staff available for weekend or holiday inseminations?
7. How is confidentiality assured?

Generally donors are selected from the student or staff population near a major medical center. Many are medical students. They are paid about $50 per specimen and enter a program for the money as well as for altruistic reasons. They are generally screened through a careful genetic-history taking. Their semen must be highly fertile and will be screened for chlamydia and other venereal infections. Blood tests from the donor should rule out syphilis, hepatitis B, cytomegalovirus, and the AIDS virus (by HTLV-III test). Recent literature recommends that donors be tested for AIDS and that the semen be frozen but not used until the donor is retested with negative results three months later. This is because it can take three months for blood tests to convert to positive after exposure to the AIDS virus. If fresh semen is to be used, donors should be questioned extensively about their sexual activity prior to each donation, and microscopic examination and culture should be done on each specimen. Some specialists exclude any donor from a program if his or his sexual partner have had *any* of the following: a blood transfusion within the year, a history of homosexual activity, multiple sexual partners, or a history of herpes.

The couple that enter an AID program will be paired with a donor who resembles the husband in coloring, height, and any other characteristics the couple specify. Some couples prefer a certain religion or ethnic group. It is very important that only one donor be used per cycle (if several have been selected) so that the paternity of the offspring will be traceable, if necessary, by the doctor. Also, mixing husband and donor semen is never an acceptable practice as it only feeds into denial of the infertility situation. It also has a detrimental affect on the chance for conception. However, most programs will permit the couple to have normal intercourse, if they wish, after an insemination.

The debate between fresh versus frozen semen still goes on, and there is little evidence that one is clearly superior to the other. Fresh semen appears to give a higher pregnancy rate, since not all sperm cells survive the freeze-thaw process. Frozen semen allows time for screening the donor more carefully. Generally two inseminations are done a month just prior to expected time of ovulation as indicated by the woman's basal temperature charts and her LH level seen in blood or urine testing. The inseminations are usually several days apart. Sometimes a third insemination is done in a cycle, but this is not usual and increases the expense and time commitment of the couple. Not all clinics are staffed on weekends or holidays, and they may not be able to provide inseminations on certain days.

The expense of AID will vary from clinic to clinic, but generally runs about $100 per office visit plus $50 per semen specimen. The cost of the blood tests and semen tests of the donor may also be charged to the couple and may amount to $200 or more. Insurance does not cover AID expenses per se, and confidentiality precludes submitting forms with the couple's name. Some doctors call the office visit a "treatment" so that the couple may attempt to recover some of their expenses.

Confidentiality of the couple is extremely important to any AID program. Complete anonymity of the donor from the couple is also very important. Most doctors keep records of the donors so that they may be retrieved if a child of AID is born with a genetic or medical problem requiring additional information. Once the woman conceives, she will be transferred to a regular obstetrician who will have no knowledge of the AID procedure. When the child is born, the father's name is entered on the birth certificate along with the mother's. The couple will need to decide if they are going to tell their child of his or her origins, and if so, when.

Prior to beginning insemination, a woman should chart her temperature for at least two to three months to become acquainted with her ovulation pattern. She will be given a pelvic exam and in some practices she will need to have a hysterosalpingogram to show that her fallopian tubes are open. Other doctors reserve the hysterosalpingogram for women who have not conceived after three or four cycles of AID. If ovulation seems regular and cervical mucus looks good, no other tests are done at this point. Some clinics are now using dip sticks in urine to test for the LH hormonal surge that occurs just prior to ovulation.

When it appears that ovulation is imminent, the woman comes to the office for the insemination. If frozen semen is used, the vial has been thawed; if fresh semen is used, the donor has left a masturbated specimen within an hour of the office visit. The semen is drawn into a small syringe and a soft rubber catheter is attached to the syringe and gently placed at the cervical opening. (If interuterine insemination is being done, the semen must be "washed" first.) A small cervical cap or tampon may be inserted to keep the semen next to the cervix. This is left in place 4 to 6 hours and the woman usually lies still on her back for 15 to 20 minutes after the insemination to help the sperm move up into the uterus and tubes. Many husbands come along for inseminations and stay with their wives throughout the procedure and the wait afterward.

It often takes at least three cycles before a pregnancy occurs. Success rates vary from 60 to 80 percent, being better for women under thirty. Exact timing is critical and this is often a problem if the woman ovulates irregularly or the clinic is not open on the day she needs to be seen. If no pregnancy has occurred after three cycles, the doctor often does a further evaluation of the wife. He might want to do a hysterosalpingogram if one hasn't been done, or a laparoscopy to rule out adhesions or endometriosis; screen for ureaplasma; or evaluate the luteal phase of the cycle via endometrial biopsy and/or plasma progesterone levels in the blood. If a problem is found, it is treated before inseminations resume.

Emotional Reactions to Donor Insemination

The couple considering AID have many feelings, which are often ambivalent. It is common for them to be at different places in readiness as well. This may lead to frustration as they consider this very logical way to have a baby (intellectually) and have entirely mixed feelings (emotionally). Coming to a point of mutual readiness and comfort may take quite a while and the help of a good counselor. Many AID programs screen the patients with a social worker for readiness to begin. For some couples, the decision is that AID will not work for both of them and relief is often felt when they can agree to try adoption or childfree living instead.

To illustrate some of the common feelings surrounding AID, conception, and birth, one sensitive case history will be quoted in its entirety. It may or may not be a typical story, but it shows how one couple felt.

My husband had an extremely low sperm count. There were many tears in the beginning. He found a doctor who prescribed several new drugs, and our hopes renewed for a while. Finally we sensed the futility of continuing with this experimental treatment and sought one final opinion elsewhere. After one simple semen analysis we were advised that we had two alternatives—adoption or AID. It didn't hit us too hard; in fact we were really relieved to be at the end of searching for cures.

Adoption seemed like such a long and difficult process and we were ready to have children right away. We didn't know much about AID, but the doctor and clinical psychologist helped us learn about it. My husband agreed that AID was the solution to our infertility. He knew I had a very strong desire to experience pregnancy. We knew it had to be something we both wanted without reservations. For three months we postponed our beginning preparations for AID. These were months of turmoil within ourselves and within our marriage. Without actually saying to my husband, "Hurry up—it's up to you," I was becoming impatient, and we both knew why.

He finally agreed to set up a preliminary appointment. At that visit we were told all about the clinic's procedure and were given physicals, and I was given some temperature charts to take for three months. We talked quite freely about what we were going through. My husband was still sensitive about his infertility, but he wanted children and wanted me to have a pregnancy. During this time I learned to appreciate my husband more and love him more deeply than I had ever thought possible. Our marriage became stronger, and sexually we grew closer and more responsive. We looked forward to the possibility of a baby. In April we were to begin our AID. The night before we were to go, we got cold feet. There were so many questions! The donor—What did he look like? What kind of person would donate sperm? How close a match would they do? The whole thing became emotional again. We were frightened when really faced with it. We were up all night trying to sort out our feelings. Finally I asked my husband if he would like more time, and he said yes. So we postponed our AID a month and hashed our many of our problems and concerns with the doctor, who was most supportive and understanding.

In May we began. I was so nervous on the first day of insemination that I lay on the table shaking. I thought I might faint for a minute. I couldn't explain my feelings of knowing that the sperm of someone whom I would never meet was inside me. All day I thought, "It's only a clinical procedure. I must think of the sperm as medicine to help me become pregnant." The second day I was not as nervous, in fact, I was quite excited. All the way back to work I was saying, "Swim, little sperm, make a baby!" I guess they heard me, as I became pregnant on the first cycle of insemination.

My husband's reaction was one of amazement and love. If it ever bothered him, he did not show it then. I had a wonderful pregnancy, feeling great physically and emotionally. I often wondered what the baby would look like. I was afraid he might not resemble either of us and people would say, "Where did you get *him?*" I also wondered whether or not my husband would accept the baby as our own. As my due date approached, we both became a little anxious. My husband was very quiet and unable to sleep well. His reason was "I've never been a father before," but I'm sure he was doing some very *heavy* thinking. . . .

Labor and delivery were a wonderful experience for both of us, and the joy we shared was the same as any couple witnessing the birth of their child. We both laughed and cried with happiness. My husband looked at our new son with love in his eyes. He kept saying, "It's amazing." Then as he hugged me, I could feel his heart pounding and I knew everything was OK. The baby was "ours" regardless of his beginning.

Artificial insemination by donor, for couples who can accept it, is an alternative growing in acceptance and popularity and regulated by medical-legal ethics. It assures the couple who are successful of not only an infant that resembles them but also the experience of a pregnancy, the chance to offer the growing baby the best possible prenatal care, and the woman the experience of labor and delivery and the chance to breast-feed. That the outcome is most often positive in every way is attested to by the number of couples who return for one or more repeat AID babies.

SURROGATE MOTHERHOOD

Of all the new technologies, surrogate motherhood is the least complicated from a technical point of view and the most controversial from an ethical or legal point of view. Surrogate motherhood is not even new. With the minor substitution of natural intercourse for artificial insemination, this can be quoted out of the Bible:

> Now Sarah, Abraham's wife, bore him no children. She had an Egyptian maid whose name was Hagar. And Sarah said to Abraham, "Behold now, the Lord has prevented me from bearing children. Go in to my maid; it may be that I shall obtain children by her." (Genesis 16:1–3)

Surrogate motherhood involves a contractual relationship between a couple desiring a child but unable to conceive because of an infertility problem of the wife or both husband and wife, and a fertile woman who is willing to bear a child for them. Surrogate programs have proliferated in the past five years and are generally for-profit businesses which solicit potential surrogates and match these surrogates with infertile couples who come to them. They may also provide medical services such as an insemination of the surrogate and provision of her prenatal, delivery, and postpartum care. They may provide legal counsel to the couple and counseling services for emotional needs. For these services, a total fee of $25,000 to $50,000 or more may be charged. From this fee, the surrogate is paid about $10,000. Since it is illegal to "buy" a baby in most states, this payment is for her *service* to the couple. Generally she is paid half the amount upon becoming successfully pregnant and the balance upon surrendering the baby to the couple.

The surrogate motherhood procedure is very simple. A surrogate is generally selected who is close to the wife in physical coloring and stature, and who may satisfy any other special requests that a couple make. Some couples feel strongly about educational background or an ethnic background. Some feel best if the woman has produced other children so they can see pictures of her progeny. The majority of women entering surrogate programs are married or have borne children. Many admit that they are doing it for the money involved, although some have an altruistic wish to help infertile couples or are women who enjoy pregnancy but have all the children they want. Once the woman has been selected, she is screened for basic health and her background on genetic diseases.

One major question in this procedure is whether the infertile couple ought to meet and interact with the surrogate, or whether anonymity should be preserved. Cases exist where the couple and the surrogate have become extremely close, to the point of the couple being present in the delivery room and receiving the newborn baby directly into their arms. Some surrogates have kept in touch after surrendering the baby and have visited. Legal and ethical concerns could arise if a surrogate *demanded* visitation rights, and, conversely, a couple could harass a surrogate who failed to surrender her baby, if they knew each other's identity and location.

Once the surrogate is selected, screened, and under contractual agreement, all that remains is for her to be inseminated during her fertile time of month, either with semen of the husband or a donor. It is imperative that the surrogate has avoided other sexual relationships in this cycle. Already one case has occurred where a baby was born deformed and, upon testing, proved to be fathered by a person other than the donor the birth-mother contracted with. This led to a lawsuit where the surrogate sued for child support for her retarded child, whom she claimed, she would never have carried to term if she had suspected to be defective. The baby lay unclaimed for months while a heartbroken couple and distraught surrogate wrangled in courts of law. There were clearly no winners here except lawyers.

Once the surrogate is pregnant, all there is left to do is wait nine months and hope for the best. In cases where the surrogate miscarries or has a stillbirth, the couple may withhold their second payment, but they do not receive a refund on the first half nor on the services already provided by the surrogate program. The contract usually spells out the policy in any of these eventualities. To this point in time, there have not been any cases of surrogate death or impairment as a result of pregnancy or delivery.

In adoption law it is not legal or binding for any woman to surrender a baby she is carrying during her pregnancy, nor is it legal for her to sign papers within several days postpartum. These laws correct a great misjustice of earlier times when young women were often coerced into surrendering a baby for adoption while they lay laboring or in the vulnerable days of their recovery. Informed consent requires that a woman be fully aware of what she is doing and signing. This law, which corrects an old abuse in adoption, now complicates surrogate motherhood, for the surrogate is, in fact, signing a contract prior to her giving birth that *requires* her to surrender her baby.

Most of the cases that have been contested in surrogate motherhood have resulted from the failure of the surrogate to surrender her baby to the couple.

Reasons given are similar: a change of heart, a feeling of bonding to the baby, or social and family pressure to keep the baby. The only recourse the couple has is to file suit for custody on the basis that the husband is the natural father and has a right to the baby just as the surrogate does. This is not possible when donor semen has been used. In the now famous *Baby M* case of Elizabeth and William Stern (would-be parents) and Mary Beth Whitehead (surrogate), Bergen County, New Jersey, Superior Court Judge Harvey Sorkow ruled that the contract signed by the surrogate was valid and upheld the awarding of custody to the father. The case is being appealed to a higher court and many family-law analysts believe the contract will be overturned at the higher level, even though custody is not expected to revert to the surrogate due to the welfare of the child. While the outcome of this case will only have legality in the state of New Jersey, it tends to give credibility to surrogate-mother programs and may have an encouraging effect in other states.

Because of the ethical and legal questions surrounding surrogate parenthood, RESOLVE has taken a cautious stance from the beginning, urging its members to explore every other medical and surgical option first, including the other new technologies of IVF, GIFT, and embryo transfer. Even adoption is seen as a preferable route, since it is protected by law in every state. If a couple decide to continue, they are well advised to have their own legal representation outside of a surrogate program to ensure that their best interests, and not just the interests of the surrogate and program, are served. An excellent discussion of surrogate motherhood and the legal ramifications can be found in *New Conceptions* by Lori B. Andrews,* who is a lawyer. RESOLVE has available the names of surrogate programs for couples who wish to explore this alternative.

CHILDFREE LIVING

One alternative available to all infertile couples and often overlooked is the right to reconsider their objective of pregnancy and parenting and to decide to remain childfree. The difference between the words *childless* and *childfree* is vast. The first connotes a negative state, something that is lacking. The second connotes a positive state, an affirmation that there can be a valuable and productive life for a couple without children.

A recent cover story in *Newsweek* magazine discussed in depth the childfree couple and the reasons for their choice. Today 1 in 4 ever-married women between the ages of twenty-five and thirty-four have never had a child—a total

---

* Lori B. Andrews, *New Conceptions* (New York: St. Martin's Press, 1984).

of nearly 3.3 million women—compared to 1 in 10 in 1960.* While some may go on to have babies after thirty-five (many say they just haven't gotten around to it), it seems clear that conscious choice for childfree living has never been more in vogue.

Sometimes the effort to achieve a pregnancy and the frustration in reaching the goal of parenting after infertility make a couple lose sight of what their motivations were in the first place. As mentioned in chapter 9, many of the forces that pressure people to have babies are externally imposed upon their value systems. They may find they are trying to make a baby not for themselves, but for society or for their parents or for their peer group, who are pressuring them to conform. One benefit of infertility (if one can find anything positive in such a crisis) is that it gives the couple a chance to reexamine their motives and assess their own needs. One conclusion they may come up with is that pregnancy and parenting is not worth the price it is extracting from their relationship. They may come to realize it isn't a personal goal or value they are really interested in. Couples who come to this realization often give up the quest for children and embark on a life that calls the *couple* a family unit and allows them to find their generativity, rewards, and fulfillment in other ways than childbearing and child rearing.

A very real help to this position was the formation of an organization called National Organization for Nonparents, founded by the articulate and often controversial Ellen Peck. In her books, *The Baby Trap* and *Pronatalism: The Myth of Mom and Apple Pie*, Ms. Peck makes some excellent revelations about forces that compel even marginally motivated people to think they have to be parents. Under suggested readings, the reader will find a number of excellent books and articles that explore whether "childfree by choice" is a workable choice for them. The trend toward remaining childfree is still a minority position and still receives renunciation from some religions and society in general. But it continues to grow.

Childfree couples can involve children in their lives in many imaginative and helpful ways in their community. Big sister and brother programs are constantly in need of a caring adult to spend quality time with a youngster in need. Volunteer coaches for girls' or boys' sports are always in demand. Teaching Sunday School can be an investment that reaps many rewards. Many couples "adopt" a niece or nephew several times a year to allow a sibling to have a much needed vacation. The possibilities are everywhere. World population no longer demands that each couple make their own children. They can share, borrow, or teach a child instead. And if they choose, they can do none of these things and yet derive good feelings of

* "Three's a Crowd," *Newsweek*, September 1, 1986, p. 68.

generativity from having creative ideas and carrying them out. The infertile couple should realize that they have the right, at any point in their investigation or treatment, to give up the quest and opt for a life not centered on children. An increasing number of couples who find AID or surrogate motherhood unacceptable and who find adoption too difficult are rethinking their values and life goals and accepting a life that is childfree.

15. Surviving Infertility

> Moon-In-The-Water . . .
> Broken-Again . . .
> Broken-Again . . .
> Still a Solid Seal.

> CHOSU

*M*any thoughts, suggestions, pieces of anecdotal material, and insights were left over when all else was carefully ordered into the chapters of this book. This last chapter is a potpourri—some observations on what hurts infertile couples, what helps them, and, reaching the ultimate goal, with children or without, how to survive infertility.

COMMENTS FROM FAMILY AND FRIENDS

Without question, the most common complaint heard from infertile couples is that people all about them are poking, probing, and pressuring them to begin a family. Remarks, often very direct and personal, are usually endured until a point of pain is reached where the couple react angrily, or withdraw in silence with their secret of infertility.

My friends and family seemed angry with us for not producing children. My mother said one Christmas, "Are you going to have a tree?" implying that two people are not sufficient to justify common traditions being carried out. A

161

woman at the country club told me I was a "cop-out" for not having children.
Another high-school friend said to me one day, "Who are you going to hug—a
dollar bill?"

Why do infertile people feel they have to endure such insensitive comments? If
they keep their infertility secret, or if they honestly give up on people by
believing "they just wouldn't understand," then the infertile couple are
unwittingly setting themselves up for one painful encounter after another—or
worse, total isolation from family and friends in an effort to be "safe."

What helps is realizing that people should be made *accountable* for their
remarks. This can be expected only if the disclosure of infertility is made. It
can be enforced only if limits are set on what family and friends have a right
to ask about. For example, one woman kept getting calls from her mother,
who lived across the country, asking, "Are you pregnant yet?" (or in more
subtle forms—"Any news?" "How *are* you?"). The woman finally told her
mother this was making her very unhappy and said that she would call *her* the
minute there was any news. Calls could continue, but the subject of
pregnancy was off limits. A person with a problem—any problem—unfortunately has the burden of explaining to others the nature of the problem, and
how others may be helpful.

I approached an intersection where a blind boy of about eighteen was
attempting to cross a busy street. I came to his side and put my hand lightly on
his shoulder and said, "Would you like me to help you across the street?" He
answered with such confidence that I was taken aback. He said, "Yes, if you will
just take a firm grip on my elbow here and tell me when we reach the opposite
curb, I would be very appreciative." After I left him at the other side I thought
for a long while about this encounter. I realized that he had helped *me* to help
him, in a way that made us both feel good. I think this is the same with infertility, but more difficult, as our problem is invisible. We have to help others to
help us.

One risk in talking openly about infertility is becoming an object of *pity*
instead of receiving the hoped-for support and understanding. No one likes to
feel pitiful. Pity places the people involved on very unequal footing. It helps
if the person who is the recipient of pity is able to explain to the offender that
pity does not comfort, it hurts. *Sympathy*, on the other hand, acknowledges
an equality of status even though there is expressed sadness and caring for the
person who is in pain.

There is no reason that infertile couples have to attend events they know in
advance will be filled with painful potential. Christenings, baby showers,
family gatherings with small children present—all have such loaded agendas
that the couple might choose to absent themselves. In time, with resolution

of the infertility problem and the feelings that accompany it, these situations will again become bearable, even enjoyable.

Although most people would not hurt another intentionally, occasionally the infertile person runs into someone who will use this subject to "one up" them or be malicious. There are also some people who, like racists and sexists, are hopeless cases for education. These people are probably best avoided.

> We had two adopted children and were awaiting a third. I was at a party and met the father of the hostess (who had four children). He asked if we had any children and I said, "We have two and another coming very soon." He stared at my tummy and realized I meant we had adopted. He shook his head and said, "I hope you'll have one of your *own* one day." I explained patiently that my adopted children *were* my own. He shook his head and said, "Well, it's nice you feel that way, but there is something special about the ones you make yourself." I stood boiling inside and considered taking this old guy really to task . . . when the absurdity of his statement made it clear he was beyond salvage. I just laughed and said, "Well, that is *one* way of looking at it."

If family and friends of infertile couples really wish to help, they should let the couple know they are available to *listen*. They should refrain from unsolicited advice and educate themselves on the subject enough to be knowledgeable—not so they can offer suggestions, but so they can understand what the couple is going through, physically and emotionally. One admission that seems to help, especially if the friends have children, is that they *cannot possibly know how it feels to be infertile*, but that they care very much about hearing the couple tell them *what they wish to tell them*. They do not poke or probe, but simply make themselves available. Their genuine love and concern will be best communicated in this kind of sharing.

PROFESSIONALS AND THE INFERTILE COUPLE

In the full course of investigation and attempted treatment of infertility, and the possible selection of an alternative, the infertile couple comes in contact with a myriad of professionals: doctors, nurses, technicians, counselors, adoption workers, and so forth. The attitudes of these people can be either very helpful or very painful. The two professions most likely to trigger reactions, partly because they wield so much potential power, are doctors and adoption workers.

The most common complaint about doctors is that they are often very rushed and seem to have little time for answering questions or offering emotional support.

He is the only doctor I know who can do a pelvic exam with one foot out the door. The fact that he is prestigious and only takes a few new cases makes me feel I cannot call him or demand anything more than what he gives me. I saw him on a local TV talk show discussing "surrogate mothers" while I was home recovering from a laparoscopy!

Here are a few pointers for the couple trying to get more time and attention from their doctor. It helps for the couple to present themselves as a team. It helps to bring an actual list of questions and concerns for discussion at the time of an appointment. It helps to ask the doctor to arrange a time to talk before or after any physical procedures *in the office*. Under no circumstances should a woman try to discuss or negotiate her case while undergoing tests or treatments in the examination room. If the end result is still a hurried and unsupportive approach, the couple is well advised to look for another doctor.

Here are a few helpful things some doctors are doing in an effort to help their patients: They are willing to see them together for a long initial visit in the office to discuss the case fully and jointly plan the goals for the future; many doctors now have a nurse counselor or social worker on their staff to offer support and information sessions, or in-depth counseling if needed; doctors are recognizing the need for telephone call-in time—such as many pediatricians offer—so that small troubles or questions can be aired without a needless office visit. Finally, more doctors than ever before are referring their patients to infertility support groups in their community, such as RESOLVE, where they can talk with others who are infertile.

Adoption workers are a close second to doctors in receiving criticism of their way of dealing with a couple in crisis, either at the initial inquiry into adoption or in the home study. *Initial inquiry* is often made so close on the heels of some bad news from the doctor that the couple are almost always still reeling and spinning and in a state of shock. The person who answers the phone inquiries at most agencies is often a receptionist. It hurts terribly if this person (whom they may mistake for an adoption worker) curtly tells them there is no waiting list, or that the list is more than five years long. What is helpful is if the initial inquiry can be passed along to a crisis counselor who can talk with the person a little more at length, commiserate on the small supply of local infants, suggest alternate types of adoption (such as legal risk or international), and invite the couple in to a general information session. These are held by many agencies every few months to deal with the many new inquiries they receive. Here couples can see other couples like themselves. They can ask questions. They can have a sense of being supported and served instead of shut out.

If the couple are able to progress to a waiting list and eventually to a home study, they may again come up with problems if the adoption worker is insensitive or threatening.

She asked us about our infertility very suddenly and abruptly after a question on something else. As I started to talk, my voice cracked and my eyes filled with tears. I was proceeding well with the story of our problems, it was just *painful*. She picked right up on my tears and said, "It looks as if you still have a lot of work to do to resolve your feelings." This made me scared and then I really did start to cry. She turned to my husband and suggested that I was too upset to continue and that we should go home and "work our feelings through" on this subject.

The home study is often a time of turmoil when old "resolved" feelings get reactivated or feelings previously unacknowledged come into view. It is the ideal time for therapeutic intervention if the adoption worker can see himself or herself as an advocate of both the child the agency will place and the family that is going to receive the child. Too often an adversarial relationship is laid down on the first encounter, where the couple feel they have to measure up to impeccable standards to *deserve* a baby, and the worker feels compelled to ferret out all the couple's deepest, darkest secrets. The most nonthreatening approach an adoption worker can use is that of being a *facilitator*. Faced with education about the adoption process and some questions about their feelings about adoption, most couples with dubious motivation select themselves out or choose to wait for a point of readiness to be achieved through counseling. The vast majority of couples entering a home study are acceptable candidates.

COUPLE COPING TECHNIQUES

In recent years whole books have been written on the subject of communications between the partners in a relationship. Many churches and counseling centers run "retreats" for couples to do intensive work on their marriages. Infertile couples often mistakenly think their only problem is infertility. For many couples, just as with any other crisis or life change, the issue is often how they are communicating with each other. This is especially important with a situation like infertility, because (1) it is a problem *both members of a couple have*, even though one may carry the burden of the diagnosis, and (2) it involves sexual and personal issues and is a lot harder to share outside the marriage with a social support system. The members may lean on one another exclusively for support, and the results may be difficult.

It is common among infertile couples for the woman to be the much more verbal and emotional partner, even if the diagnosis is a male factor. One RESOLVE counselor, Merle Bombardieri, suggests use of the "20-minute rule" to help keep infertility from becoming an all-consuming event and to break the pattern of lopsided communications. She suggests the couple set aside a period of time each evening to talk about infertility. Using a timer to limit each person to 20 minutes, first one speaks and then the other. The person not speaking is asked to listen intently. This technique is particularly helpful in achieving these outcomes:

1. The wife will talk less about infertility and will present her feelings more succinctly.
2. The husband is more willing to listen because he is assured of an end point.
3. The wife feels she has an interested listener and is supported.
4. Both may feel relieved to see the other feeling better.
5. Then the rest of the evening may be spent in more pleasant pursuits.
6. In all likelihood, as the wife feels she has less need to talk about infertility, the husband will begin to do more. Bombardieri notes that in many cases she has seen, the wife has actually been "grieving for two."*

Couple support groups are another excellent way for couples to cope with the infertility experience. Often what they have been unable to hear from a spouse, they can hear and accept from another group member. At first, members of a group are very oriented to "who has the problem" within each couple, and they are very polarized by sex—that is, the women support the women and the men support the men. Later on in a group's process, one sees transferences to like issues in a member of the opposite sex, that is, "We are both the infertile members in our marriages," and surprising support for characteristics, traits, and situations that are similar in opposite-sex members, that is, "I'm just like you; I have no family to share this with." One of the healthiest things that happens in a well-run group is confrontation by one member of another, often over an issue of marital communications. A group member can usually accept this from another member better than from a spouse. The leader is present to be sure that confrontations are fair and not one-sided. The other group members and the leader lend an objectivity to a relationship, which is very helpful.

An excellent book by a RESOLVE member and family therapist includes exercises and anecdotal material that is very useful to the couple struggling in their communications; this is Linda Salzar's *Infertility: How Couples Can Cope* (see the bibliography for this and other helpful resources).

RELIGION AND FAITH

Formal religion may be a source of pressure (to produce children) and even guilt about how the couple may choose to go about overcoming their

---

* Merle Bombardieri, "The Twenty Minute Rule: First Aid for Couples in Distress," *RESOLVE Newsletter*, December 1983, p. 5.

infertility. Couples who are members of faiths that do not condone the "new technologies," use of donor semen, or even masturbation to obtain a semen analysis, must come to grips with both their religious convictions and their medical convictions. Sometimes the two clash; in an increasing number of cases, couples are choosing to accept their "individual conscience" to decide their course of treatment.

More commonly, religion and faith play a comforting and supportive role in the infertility struggle. Several testimonies follow:

I have a daughter who is almost six. After two and a half years of trying for a second child, I found renewed religious faith and prayed daily, "Please, God, give me another child." I could not pray, "Your will be done," as I felt another child was the only solution. I became increasingly miserable and angry. Someone told me that if God gives us something in life that is hard to handle, He also gives us the strength to handle it. I couldn't stand my miserable state, so I changed my prayer at last to "Your will be done" and felt an instant relief from my misery. I still hope to become pregnant. God allows us to have hope. But I have given my burden of infertility to the Lord and feel a sense of peace.

I believed for quite a while that God was punishing me by withholding the baby we so earnestly desired. I atoned through various painful professional and volunteer projects that brought me into daily contact with unwed mothers. Still no pregnancy. I finally talked with our minister (who was a woman) and she said "Our concept of God is not of a punishing or withholding Power. Our God is not vested with giving or taking away, but is a benevolent, all-caring Presence." She suggested that the science of medicine might conquer (or not conquer) our infertility, and that God could give us the courage, the strength, and ultimately the peace to accept our fate.

DREAMS AND FANTASIES

Some of the powerful feelings of infertility may be played out in dreams and fantasies as well as in everyday thought. These images from the deeper recesses of the mind are often recurrent and may persist long after the actual situation is resolved. Dreams and fantasies are helpful in coping with feelings of infertility and in working them through.

I have a favorite fantasy about what it would be like telling my husband I am pregnant. There is no taking of temperatures, no programmed sex, no worry about my period coming. Just one day I discover I am pregnant. I go out and have my hair done and buy a new dress (a little loose). On my way home I buy steaks and a bottle of champagne. Dinner is elegant, with candlelight and wine. We talk of his day at the office and all the other news . . . the delay in telling is what is such fun in this fantasy. Finally, lingering over coffee, gazing at him through the candles, I say, "I have something to tell you, Jim. I'm pregnant!" He is amazed; he is thrilled! We embrace (it's just like a Doris Day movie). Bring on the champagne!

I have a crazy recurring dream that I got pregnant but that it was necessary to borrow Bob's stomach for the whole nine months!

When I was in the midst of my infertility workup, I began dreaming about giving birth. These were no small dreams—they were gigantic Cecil B. DeMille productions with casts of thousands. I was always at the center, very beautiful and in control. My husband was standing at my side and I labored (sweating ever so slightly) briefly, then had a wonderful birth. The baby was perfect and everyone cheered and praised me for how well I had done. My husband was crying and telling me how much he loved me. Once I awoke in the middle of this dream (which recurred for years) and I found myself with my legs drawn up and bearing down as if I were really giving birth!

We've created such an absurd fantasy in our minds as to what life with a child would be like that it could never possibly meet our expectations. I imagine a smiling and happy baby—always immaculate—with my husband and me beaming proudly, completely contented, with few worries. Life is beautiful and we feel fulfilled. I visualize a lovely little girl with blond hair and blue eyes, dressed in yards and yards of ribbon and lace. . . .

One common theme to most dreams and fantasies is sense of control and mastery over situations that the infertile person has so often lost in reality. In this sense, and as an outlet for otherwise repressed fears and feelings, dreams and fantasies are no doubt helpful.

ANIMALS AND OTHER LIVING THINGS

A universal outlet for the longing to nurture felt by the infertile couple is given to pets and growing things. Most commonly the nurturance is transferred to a lovable and furry pet such as a dog or cat, which gives great satisfaction in return. But couples report pleasure in almost anything alive, from tropical fish to horses to gardens.

We could not have pets in our apartment, which made me very sad. I had never had much luck with plants, but I proceeded to buy an enormous number of African violets and a fluorescent light unit to grow them under. I mixed superfertile soil for potting; I fed them extra nutrients each week. I was rewarded with brilliant blossoms. Each plant took on a character of its own. If one damped off and died I felt a great loss; those which were richest in display were centerpieces for our table. I don't know what Freud would make of my several years of plant fetish, but it gave me a feeling of control over fertility—and something *alive* that I could call my own.

It is common for pet owners to ascribe human thoughts and feelings to their animal friends For the infertile couple this can manifest itself in treating pets as children and in enjoying the extra time and attention they require, and also in complaining (though not too bitterly) over their mishaps and accidents. Some couples carry photos of their pets to have something to show when fertile couples are showing their photos of children. One obviously loaded area in regard to pets is their fertility.

> I got this adorable female kitten at the local humane society. I knew from the start I wanted a female, though I hadn't given much thought to why. When she neared six months of age I asked the vet about the best time to spay her. He recommended doing it at once, since many female cats, once they mature, are literally never out of heat long enough to have the operation. I thought about letting her have one litter, but I also believed firmly that wanton breeding of cats and dogs is immoral. How I struggled with the decision to have her fixed! I should explain that I had recently had ovarian surgery myself and my outlook was very dim. I looked at her eyes and they seemed to be pleading with me to let her be a mother *just once!* The event that decided things in a hurry was her first heat. She was unbearable! I took her right in for her operation after that. Afterward, I often thought she looked at me with a look that had special meaning between us. I would stroke her and say, "We're just a couple of spayed cats, huh, Goldie?"

Some people raise valuable animals and breed for stud. There is probably a vicarious thrill in the successful mating and rearing of animals when personal fertility is denied. This may lead some to let dogs and cats of no particular value breed at will, forcing many offspring into poor homes or the certain death of a humane society ward.

The death of a beloved pet, for anyone, may be very traumatic. If that pet was considered as a surrogate child for the couple, the grief may equal the intensity of the loss of a child. Once again, society will negate such grief and the couple are often very private with their feelings. Since pets and other growing things are valuable as objects of nurturance, it is also very painful when that beloved object is lost.

TIME

"The trouble with time is that . . . *it takes so long!*" This is an often heard protest when infertile couples are consoled with the fact that they will feel better by and by. It is true that the passage of time heals. It is also true that it can't be hurried or telescoped. Time seems to bring with it a sense of *perspective* or "the larger view" of life for those who have had tunnel vision focused on infertility for a number of years. When feelings have been properly worked through, they tend to subside and a kind of *selective remembering* often takes place so that the really painful memories and events are muted. Time is a healer, time is a friend. But *time takes time.*

THE ROLE OF HUMOR

In the face of adversity, laughter is indeed the best medicine. It helps enormously if a couple can keep their sense of perspective and their sense of humor enough to indulge in occasional laughter at the absurdity of some of the situations infertility imposes upon them. RESOLVE support groups often begin with a great deal of anger and upset, so-called war stories of what the couples are going through, and they almost invariably are characterized by increasing amounts of banter and laughter as therapy progresses. This reflects the willingness to let go of some of the control of a frequently uncontrollable situation, and the ability to not take oneself too seriously in the face of adversity. Some of the "jokes" in support groups are so subtle that only infertile people would understand them. Here are some examples from anecdotes sent to RESOLVE or shared in support groups.

> All of the waiting, the painfully slow cycles due to having to wait for bodily processes to run their course, made us realize how totally out of control we were. Because of the methodical plodding along, we came to refer to ourselves as "infertile turtles." We could think of nothing more appropriate. Turtledom was a very isolating experience. We never told anyone of our animal identities. We even had a theme song. There was a song from *Cabaret* called "Maybe This Time" and with a few changes the song became "Maybe This Month."

> I was delivering my husband's 24-hour urine specimen in a large jar in a big brown bag. The hospital was located in a high-crime area of town and I suppose I was clutching the bag to my body. A man came out of nowhere and grabbed the bag away from me. I was just dumbfounded! Several people came to my assistance and I just began to laugh until I cried and I couldn't get a word out.

> I will never forget a talk show interview I did on infertility while in Nashville. This really suave and debonair male host (on live TV) looked at me and asked, "Is infertility usually a hereditary problem?" I had all I could do to keep my composure. "No. . . ," I started thoughtfully. "I think we can say with certainty that absolute infertility is *never* hereditary."

My husband had to take a six-month training course at the exact time the doctor decided to put me on fertility pills. His schedule was crazy—two weeks in New York, three weeks in Atlanta, one week in Buffalo, and so on. We were still relative newlyweds (married two years) and no one knew about the fertility pills. All they did know was that my husband had one very impassioned wife who followed him all over the country while all the other wives stayed at home. It got to be a joke with us—"Have thermometer, will travel!"

Our support group got into this really hilarious discussion about what sort of container makes the ideal vessel to deliver a semen specimen. We all agreed that 5 cc of semen in a mayonnaise jar looks too pathetic to even consider. On the other hand, our wives' empty perfume bottles were virtually impossible to hit and were somewhat effeminate. Used caviar jars or artichoke heart jars were just the right size, but we felt "pretentious." We finally agreed that the ideal jar to deliver a semen specimen in was that one item an infertile couple would never have in the house—an empty baby food jar.

The humor of infertility is often wry and low-key. There aren't too many sidesplitters when it comes to this problem. Humor adds levity to an otherwise depressing situation. It adds balance and perspective to stressful and frustrating situations. Those who can see humor in the midst of their travail are most blessed.

CONTACT WITH OTHER INFERTILE COUPLES

No one understands infertility as well as someone who has been there. Finding another person or couple who are experiencing infertility may be easy for some who are candid and open about their own situation. But many couples honestly do not know one other man or woman who is or ever has been infertile. *This in a country where more than 10 million people are currently infertile!* It could be their next-door neighbor, the man who manages the local gas station, the woman at the local library reference desk— almost anyone with no children. The problem is that *infertility does not show*. And to presume lack of children is equal to infertility is frequently wrong. Infertile people simply have no way of finding one another without help.

RESOLVE was founded in Boston in 1973 for exactly that reason. A small group of women who were experiencing infertility "found one another" at an adoption conference and decided to hold monthly discussions about what they were feeling. The idea was so successful that soon the group expanded and increased to weekly meetings and the depth of a true support group. Later came a telephone counseling service staffed by a volunteer nurse. Still later came a small newsletter to send to our increasing membership. The call came from other cities and other states for services in their areas. RESOLVE, which is nonprofit and charitable, has now expanded to a national organization with more than 40 chapters and a membership in the thousands. Fact sheets, reprints of good articles, suggested reading lists, and other resources are available to members as well as an excellent national newsletter published five times a year. Through this clearinghouse, members can be put in contact with others in their area who are infertile. They can join support groups and attend conferences. They can discover that they are not alone and help educate themselves to receive the best possible medical care. The organization also helps couples who are turning to alternatives such as adoption, donor insemination, or childfree living. Contact with other infertile couples is one of the most helpful ways to break through the isolation and despair of the infertility experience. Information on joining RESOLVE is found in the section on organizations and resources.

CONCLUSION

In spite of medical advances and "new technologies," there has never been a harder time to be infertile. The 10 million Americans whose lives and hopes are touched by infertility are caught between two opposite and powerful social currents. The first is the traditional value system of religion, family, and culture that says marriage and childbearing are expected duties of the adult person. The other is the social trend toward zero population growth, childfree marriages, and the dissolution of family values. In the eyes of the first segment of the population, the infertile couple are seen as objects of pity or even scorn. In the eyes of the second, infertility may be seen as a "blessing" or, at worst, a minor inconvenience. People who work at achieving pregnancy in a time of world overpopulation have even been called "immoral."

The decisions on medical and surgical procedures to overcome infertility have never been more complicated. Some, such as in vitro, donor insemination, and surrogate mothering involve ethical, legal, and moral dilemmas as well. If the couple cannot be helped by science, and half of all cases cannot, the alternative of an adoptable infant is becoming less and less available.

The infertile couple deserve advocacy and respect. Theirs is a problem that is a legitimate public-health concern—one that is alarmingly on the rise in recent years. Infertility cannot remain shrouded in superstition, stigma, and misinformation if we are to help overcome it. While it rarely proves fatal or incapacitating physically, infertility exacts a heavy toll on the emotions, finances, and quality of life of those affected. A health problem affecting 10 million people cannot be denied. Its victims may be invisible, but they are joining forces and resources as never before. They will be heard. They will be helped.

Glossary

Abortion. The premature expulsion of an embryo from the uterus. When an abortion is intentional, it is known as an induced or therapeutic abortion, or termination of pregnancy. When it occurs naturally, it is known as a spontaneous abortion or a miscarriage.

Adhesion. An abnormal attachment of adjacent serous membrane bands or masses of connective tissue.

Amniocentesis. The removal of a small sample of amniotic fluid from the uterus between the fourteenth and sixteenth week of pregnancy for chromosome analysis. Used primarily in women over thirty-five.

Amenorrhea. The absence of menstruation.

Ampulla. The widening in the upper end of the vas deferens of the male, in which some sperm are stored.

Andrology. The science of diseases of men.

Anovulation. The failure of ovulation to occur.

Anovulatory Bleeding. The type of menstruation associated with failure to ovulate. It may be scanty and of short duration or abnormally heavy, often occurring in irregular patterns. May also be called *breakthrough bleeding*.

Artificial Insemination by Donor (AID). The instillation of donor semen into the woman's vagina for purposes of conception.

Artificial Insemination by Husband (AIH). The instillation of a husband's semen into the wife's vagina for purposes of conception.

Azoospermia. The complete absence of sperm in the ejaculate.

Basal Body Temperature (BBT). The temperature of the woman taken in the morning, upon awakening, before any activity.

Bicornuate Uterus. A congenital malformation of the uterus where it is

173

divided internally to some degree by a septum and appears to have two "horns."

Biopsy. The surgical removal of tissue for analysis.

Blastocyst. A fertilized ovum that after about 5 days' development implants in the wall of the uterus.

Blighted Pregnancy. A fertilized ovum that fails to develop after implanting and aborts spontaneously.

Capacitation. The wearing away of the sperm's outer protective coating that allows the sperm to penetrate and fertilize an ovum. May occur naturally in the passage through the woman's reproductive tract or in "sperm washing" prior to certain procedures.

Cauterize. To coagulate or destroy tissue by applying heat.

Cervix. The neck or opening of the uterus into the vagina.

Chlamydia. A microorganism found in the genitourinary tract; may be transmitted by sexual contact.

Chromosome. A cell that carries the material determining hereditary characteristics.

Coitus. Sexual relations.

Conception. Pregnancy.

Congenital Defect. A characteristic present at birth, acquired during pregnancy.

Contraception. Prevention of pregnancy by any means.

Corpus Luteum. The special gland that forms in the ovary at the site of ovulation and produces the hormone progesterone in the second half of the normal menstrual cycle.

Cryptorchidism. The undescended testicles in the male.

Culdoscopy. The direct visualization of the pelvic cavity by means of an instrument inserted through a small incision in the vagina. Used prior to development of laparoscopy, which is now preferred.

Dilation and Curettage (D&C). The dilation of the cervix to allow scraping of the uterine lining with an instrument called a curette. Can be done as a therapeutic measure in infertility, or following spontaneous abortion. It is also a method of therapeutic abortion in the first trimester.

Dysmenorrhea. Painful menstruation.

Dyspareunia. Painful sexual intercourse.

Ectopic Pregnancy. A pregnancy that implants anywhere but in the uterus. Some possible sites are the fallopian tube, the ovary, or, rarely, in the abdominal cavity.

Ejaculation. The male orgasm, during which approximately 2 to 5 cubic centimeters of seminal fluid are ejected from the penis.

Embryo. An early stage of prenatal development, used until the eighth week, after which time the term *fetus* is used.

Embryo Freezing. Use of cryopreservation to preserve an embryo or embryos fertilized through in vitro or natural means and not needed in the cycle of treatment a woman is undergoing.

Embryo Transfer. Used extensively in animal husbandry, this procedure is still new in human infertility. A woman unable to produce her own ovum receives the fertilized egg (embryo) of a donor woman. It is instilled into her uterus just prior to the implantation phase. Her cycle must be synchronized hormonally with the donor.

Endocrinologist. A doctor who specializes in disease of the endocrine or hormone system.

Endometriosis. The presence of endometrial tissue (normal uterine lining) in abnormal locations, such as the fallopian tubes, the ovaries, or the peritoneal cavity. A leading cause of infertility.

Endometrial Biopsy. Extraction of a small sample of tissue from the uterine lining for examination. Usually done to show evidence of ovulation.

Endometrium. The mucous membrane lining of the uterus.

Epididymis. An elongated organ in the male scrotum lying above and behind the testicles. It contains a highly convoluted canal, 4 to 6 meters in length, where sperm are ripened and nourished and stored after production for a period of several months.

Erection. The enlarged state of the penis when aroused.

Estrogen. The primary female hormone, produced mainly in the ovaries from puberty until menopause.

Fallopian Tube. The long, narrow tube between the ovary and the uterus. After release of the egg from the ovary, the tube transports the egg to the uterus.

Fertilization. The penetration of the ovum by a sperm.

Fetus. The term applied to the unborn conceptus after 8 weeks until birth.

Fibroid Tumor. A benign tumor of fibrous tissue that may occur in the uterine wall. May exist without symptoms or may cause abnormal menstrual patterns or infertility.

Fimbriated Ends. The fringed and flaring outer ends of the fallopian tubes.

Follicle. A small sac in the ovary in which an ovum develops.

Follicular Stimulating Hormone (FSH). A hormone produced in the anterior pituitary that stimulates the ovary to ripen a follicle for ovulation.

Frigidity. The inability of the woman to become sexually aroused to the point of achieving orgasm. Not a known cause of infertility.

Fundus. The upper portion of the uterus, farthest away from the cervix.

Gamete. The male or female reproductive cells, the sperm or the ovum.

Gamete Intrafallopian Transfer (GIFT). Several ripened ova from the woman (or a donor) and a prepared semen specimen from the man (or a donor) are placed in the distal end of the fallopian tube. If fertilization takes place, it does so in the natural setting and the embryo does not require transferring to the uterus. Only used in women who have functional tubes.

Genetic. Pertaining to hereditary characteristics.

Gonadotropins. The pituitary hormones that stimulate the reproductive system.

Gonads. The glands that make the gametes, the testicles in the male and the ovaries in the female.

Gonorrhea. An infection spread by sexual contact, caused by the *Gonococcus neisseria*.

Gynecologist. A doctor who specializes in diseases of women.

Habitual Abortion. The recurrent spontaneous loss of a fetus.

Hemorrhage. Uncontrolled bleeding.

Hirsutism. Excessive hairiness.

Hormone. A chemical produced by an endocrine gland in the body that circulates in the blood and has widespread action throughout the body.

Hostile Cervical Mucus. Cervical mucus that destroys or immobilizes sperm.

Hühner Test. See *Postcoital Test*.

Human Chorionic Gonadotropin (HCG). A hormone secreted by the placenta in pregnancy that prolongs the life of the corpus luteum and thus preserves the pregnancy. This hormone accounts for pregnancy tests being positive. It may be given therapeutically in some infertility problems.

Hyperplasia. An abnormal enlargement of an organ or tissue of the body.

Hypothalamus. A part of the base of the brain that controls the action of the pituitary gland.

Hysterectomy. The surgical removal of the uterus. This can be total removal of uterus and cervix or *partial*, meaning that the uterus is removed, but the cervix remains.

Hysteroscopy. The direct visualization of the interior of the uterus with an instrument called a hysteroscope. Small surgical repairs can also be done during this procedure.

Hysterotomy. The opening of the uterus surgically for purposes of removal of tumors or repair of structural problems. The uterus is then sutured closed and remains in place.

Hysterosalpingogram (HSG). An X-ray study in which radiopaque dye is injected into the uterus through the cervix to show the delineation of the body of the uterus and the patency of the fallopian tubes. Also called a *tubogram* or *uterotubogram*.

Immunologic Response. The presence of sperm antibodies in the woman or man that tend to destroy the sperm's fertility by immobilizing them or making them clump together.

Implantation. The embedding of the fertilized ovum in the endometrium of the uterus, usually on or about day 5 after fertilization.

Impotence. The inability to achieve or maintain an erection for intercourse. May be due to physical or emotional causes or a combination of both.

Infertility. The inability of a couple to achieve a pregnancy after one year of regular unprotected sexual relations, or the inability of the woman to carry a pregnancy to a live birth.

Incompetent Cervix. A cervix that dilates prematurely during pregnancy. May result in the loss of the fetus in the second trimester.

Interstitial Cells. The cells between the seminiferous tubules of the testicles that produce the male hormone testosterone. Also called *Leydig's cells.*

Intrauterine Device (IUD). A contraceptive device placed in the uterus to prevent pregnancy. No longer in common use in the United States.

In Vitro Fertilization (IVF). Fertilization of an egg and sperm that takes place outside the body in a special medium in a glass dish. The embryo(s) is then instilled into the mother's uterus just prior to the implantation phase. Also called *extracorporeal fertilization.*

Karyotype. A photograph of the arrangement of chromosomes in the nucleus of a cell. Used for genetic counseling.

Klinefelter's Syndrome. A congenital abnormality of the male wherein he receives an extra X chromosome in the sex gene, giving an XXY instead of the normal XY. Most men with this condition are sterile.

Labia Majora. The large outer lips of the vulva of the woman.

Labia Minora. The inner lips of the vulva.

Lactation. The production of milk by the glands of the breast.

Laparoscopy. The direct visualization of the pelvic organs by means of an instrument called a laparoscope. It is introduced into the pelvic cavity while the woman is under anesthesia, through a small incision near the navel. Used in diagnostic and also some minor treatment procedures.

Libido. The desire for sexual intercourse.

Luteinizing Hormone (LH). A hormone secreted by the anterior lobe of the pituitary during the entire menstrual cycle, with a "peak" just before ovulation. May be given therapeutically in infertility conditions. LH is the hormone that urine home-testing kits use to predict ovulation.

Menarche. The onset of menstruation in girls.

Menopause. The cessation of menstruation in women, because of age or failure or removal of the ovaries. Also called *the change of life.* Most commonly occurs between forty-five and fifty-five years of age. Surgical menopause is abrupt cessation of menstruation because of the removal of the ovaries or uterus and ovaries.

Menstruation. The cyclic bleeding that normally occurs about once a month in the mature female, in the absence of pregnancy, from menarche to menopause. It is the shedding of the uterine lining.

Microsurgery. The surgery performed on delicate body tissues by use of special lenses and techniques.

Miscarriage. The spontaneous abortion of a fetus up to the age of viability.

Mittleschmertz. The German word for "middle pain," it refers to pain upon ovulation that some women experience.

Motility. The ability to move, as in sperm.

Mucus. A clear secretion from any mucous membrane that keeps the membrane moist.

Myomectomy. The surgical removal of a tumor (myoma) in the muscular wall of the uterus.

Nidation. The attachment of the fertilized ovum to the endometrium of the uterus.

Obstetrician. A doctor who specializes in the management of pregnancy and childbirth.

Oligospermia. A scarcity of sperm in the ejaculate.

Oocyte. A primitive cell that becomes an ovum.

Oophorectomy. The surgical removal of an ovary.

Orchiditis. The inflammation of the testicles. Seen in cases of adult mumps.

Orgasm. The moment of sexual climax, marked by ejaculation in the male and feelings of excitement and pleasure in the female.

Ovaries. The sexual glands of the female that produce the hormones estrogen and progesterone and in which ova develop. There are two ovaries, one on each side of the uterus behind the fallopian tubes.

Ovulation. The discharge of a ripened ovum, usually at the midpoint of the menstrual cycle.

Ovum. The egg cell ripened in a follicle of the ovary once each month.

Pap Test. A simple swabbing of the cervical os to determine the presence of cancerous cells. Recommended every year or two for women over the age of twenty.

Pathologist. A doctor who specializes in examination of tissue specimens.

Pelvic Inflammatory Disease (PID). A general infection of the uterus, tubes, and peritoneal cavity which may be caused by a number of different organisms. A primary cause of infertility in women.

Pelvis. The area surrounded by the iliac bones, mons pubis, and sacrum, supported by muscle and ligaments and containing the reproductive organs of the woman as well as the bladder and intestines.

Penis. The male organ through which urine and semen are emitted.

Peritoneum. The tissue covering the inside of the abdominal wall.

Pituitary. A gland located at the base of the brain that secretes a number of important hormones related to normal growth and development and fertility.

Placenta. A spongy organ developed only during pregnancy to serve as the conductor of nutrients and oxygen to the growing fetus in utero. The fetus is connected to the placenta by the umbilical cord.

Polycystic Ovaries (PCO). A condition in which many ovarian cysts enlarge the ovaries and cause infertility. Also called *Stein-Leventhal syndrome.*

Polyp. A nodule or small growth found frequently on mucous membranes such as the cervix or uterus.

Postcoital Test. A diagnostic test of infertility wherein vaginal and cervical secretions are analyzed under a microscope within several hours of intercourse. A normal test shows large numbers of live and motile sperm. Also called the *Hühner test* or the *PK test.*

Progesterone. A hormone secreted by the corpus luteum of the ovary after ovulation has occurred. Also produced by the placenta in pregnancy.

Prolactin. A pituitary hormone that stimulates the milk glands of the breast in the female.

Prostate. A gland in the male that surrounds the first portion of the urethra, after the bladder. It secretes an alkaline liquid that neutralizes the acidity of the urethra and the vagina, and it stimulates the motility of sperm.

Pseudocyesis. Also called *false pregnancy,* a condition simulating pregnancy in which the woman believes herself to be pregnant but is not.

Puberty. The time of life when male and female reproductive organs become functional. Typically female puberty occurs earlier than male puberty.

Radiologist. A doctor who specializes in taking and interpreting X rays of the body.

Retrograde Ejaculation. The semen that backs up into the bladder instead of out of the penis upon ejaculation. Often due to neurologic problems, diabetes, or medication.

Rubin's Test. An outdated test of infertility in which carbon dioxide is blown through the cervix and escapes out the fallopian tubes if they are patent. Also called *tubal insufflation.*

Scrotum. The bag of skin and thin muscle that holds the testicles.

Secondary Infertility. The inability to conceive or carry a pregnancy after one or more successful pregnancies.

Secretory Phase. The second half of the menstrual cycle, after about day 14, when the endometrium is preparing to receive the fertilized egg.

Semen. The sperm and seminal secretions ejaculated during orgasm.

Semen Analysis. The study of the fresh ejaculation under the microscope to count the number of million sperm per cubic centimeter, to check the shape and size of the sperm, and to note their ability to move (motility).

Seminal Vesicles. A pair of pouchlike glands above the prostate in the male that produce a secretion rich in fructose, a nutrient needed by sperm to fuel their journey. Some sperm are also stored in these pouches prior to ejaculation.

Seminiferous Tubules. The long tubes in the testicles in which sperm cells are formed.

Sexually Transmitted Disease. Any infection known to be transmitted by sexual intercourse. Some common infections are gonorrhea, chlamydia, ureaplasma, syphilis, and herpes. Untreated infections are a significant cause of infertility, especially in women.

Spermatogenesis. The production of sperm within the seminiferous tubules.

Spermatozoa. The male reproductive cell. Synonymous with sperm.

Split Ejaculate. A method of collecting a semen specimen so that the first half of the ejaculate is caught in one container and the rest in a second. The first half contains the vast majority of motile sperm.

Stein-Leventhal Syndrome. See *Polycystic Ovaries*.

Surrogate Motherhood. The contracting with a woman to bear a child. She is usually inseminated with sperm of the husband of the infertile woman. The woman is paid for her services and is required to surrender the baby after birth. A controversial practice from legal and ethical points of view.

Testicle. The male sexual gland, of which there are two. They are contained in the scrotal sac. They produce the male hormone testosterone and produce the male reproductive cells, sperm.

Testicular Biopsy. A small surgical excision of testicular tissue to determine the ability of cells to produce normal sperm and the hormone testosterone.

Testosterone. The most important male sex hormone produced in the testicles.

Test-Tube Baby. A popular term for a baby conceived by in vitro fertilization.

Thyroid Gland. A gland located at the front base of the neck that secretes the hormone thyroid, found to be necessary for normal fertility.

T-Mycoplasma. A microorganism thought to be implicated in infertility and in some miscarriages. It is sexually transmitted.

Tubal Insufflation. See *Rubin's Test*.

Turner's Syndrome. A congenital abnormality of the female wherein she receives a single X instead of an XX genetic sex complement. Women with this condition have no ovarian function.

Ultrasound. A diagnostic technique that uses sound waves rather than X rays to visualize internal body structures.

Undescended Testicles. Testicles that have not descended naturally into the scrotal sac.

Urethra. The passage that carries urine from the bladder in the woman, and in the man also carries semen from the prostate gland to the point of ejaculation during intercourse.

Urologist. A doctor who specializes in diseases of the urinary tract in men and women and also the reproductive organs in men.

Uterus. The hollow, muscular organ in the woman whose specific purpose is the lodging and nourishment of the fetus until the time of birth.

Vagina. The "birth canal" of the woman, extending from the vulva upward to the cervix of the uterus.

Vaginismus. A spasm of the muscles around the opening of the vagina, making penetration during sexual intercourse either impossible or very painful. Can be organic or psychogenic in origin.

Varicocele. A varicose vein of the testicle, thought to be a significant cause of infertility in some males.

Vasa Deferentia (singular, vas deferens). A pair of thick-walled tubes, about 45 centimeters long, in the male, that lead from the epididymis to the ejaculatory duct in the prostate gland. During ejaculation, these ducts make wavelike contractions to propel the sperm forward.

Vasectomy. The surgical interruption of the vas deferens for purposes of permanent sterilization of the male.

Venereal Disease. See *Sexually Transmitted Disease.*

Vulva. The folds of skin that protect the entrance to the vagina.

Bibliography

Books on Infertility

Andrews, Lori B., *New Conceptions: A Consumer's Guide to the Newest Infertility Treatment*. New York: St. Martin's Press, 1984. (Focuses on legal aspects of the new technologies.)

Bellina, Joseph H., and Josleen Wilson, *You Can Have a Baby*, New York: Crown Publishers, 1985.

Garcia, Celso-Ramon, M.D., et al., *Current Therapies of Infertility*. St. Louis, MO: C. V. Mosby, 1984.

Lipshultz, Larry I., M.D., and Stuart S. Howards, M.D., *Infertility in the Male*. New York: Churchill Livingstone, 1983.

Mason, Mary Martin, *The Miracle Seekers*. Fort Wayne, IN: Perspectives Press, 1987. (See Resources and Organizations for address. An anthology of short stories about infertility.)

Mazor, Miriam D., M.D., and Harriet F. Simon, eds., *Infertility: Medical, Emotional, and Social Considerations*. New York: Human Sciences Press, Inc., 1983.

Salzar, Linda P., *Infertility: How Couples Can Cope*. Boston: G. K. Hall Publishers, Inc., 1986.

Articles on Infertility

Clapp, Diane N., "Emotional Response to Infertility: Nursing Interventions," *Journal of Obstetrics and Gynecologic Neonatal Nursing*, 14:6, 1985.

Clark, Matt, et al., "Infertility: New Cures, New Hope," *Newsweek*, December 6, 1982, pp. 102–110.

Coman, Carolyn, "Trying (and Trying and Trying) to Get Pregnant," *Ms.*, May 1983, pp. 21–24.

Harris, Diane, "What It Costs to Fight Infertility," *Money*, December 1984, pp. 201–212.

Henig, Robin Marantz, "New Hope for Troubled Couples," *Woman's Day*, May 22, 1984, pp. 32–43.

Menning, Barbara Eck, "The Emotional Needs of Infertile Couples," *Fertility and Sterility*, 34:4, October 1980, pp. 313–319.

Quindlen, Anna, "Baby Craving, *Life*, June 1987, pp. 23–42.

Yalof, Ina, "As the Sperm Turns," *Gentleman's Quarterly*, March 1986, pp. 158–165.

General Health and Consumer Advocacy

Bluestone, Naomi, M.D., "What's Up Doc?" *Health*, March 1985, p. 76.

Boston Women's Health Book Collective, *Our Bodies, Ourselves*. New York: Simon and Schuster, 1985. (Has a chapter on infertility.)

U.S. Congress, Office of Technology Assessment, *Reproductive Health Hazards in the Workplace*. Washington, DC: U.S. Government Printing Office, 1985.

Pregnancy Loss

Adler, Jerry, et al., "Learning from the Loss," *Newsweek*, March 24, 1986, pp. 66–67.

Berezin, Nancy, *After a Loss in Pregnancy*. New York: Simon and Schuster, 1982.

Berg, Susan, and Judith Lasker, *When Pregnancy Fails: Families Coping with Miscarriage, Stillbirth, and Infant Death*. Boston: Beacon Press, 1981.

Friedman, Rochelle, M.D., and Bonnie Gradstein, *Surviving Pregnancy Loss*. Boston: Little, Brown and Co., 1982.

Page, Tim, "Life Miscarried," *New York Times Magazine*, January 27, 1985, p. 50.

Schweibert, Pat R., and Paul Kirk, M.D., *Still to Be Born*. (Order from Perinatal Loss, 2116 N.E. 18th Ave., Portland, OR 97212, $4.00.)

Special Topics

Bichler, Joyce, *DES Daughter: A True Story of Tragedy and Triumph*. New York: Avon Books, 1981.

McKaughan, Molly, "The Ectopic Epidemic," *Woman's Day*, April 3, 1984, pp. 62–65.

Morgan, Susanne, *Coping with a Hysterectomy*, New York: Dial Press, 1982.

Older, Julia, *Endometriosis*. New York: Charles Scribner's Sons, 1983.

Orenberg, Cynthia Laitman, *DES. The Complete Story*. New York: St. Martin's Press, 1981.

In Vitro Fertilization (IVF)

Blake, Jeanne, "Children of Love, Children of Science," *Boston*, December 1984, pp. 194–197.

Clapp, Diane N., and Merle Bombardieri, "Easing Stress for IVF Patients and Staff," *Contemporary Ob/Gyn*, 24:4, October 1984, pp. 91–99.

Jones, Howard W., Jr., Georgeanna Seegar Jones, Gary D. Hodgen, and Zev Rosenwaks, *In Vitro Fertilization*. Baltimore, MD: Williams and Wilkins, 1986. (Highly technical medical text about IVF.)

Phillips, Meg, "One Woman's Courage," *American Health*, November 1985, pp. 76–90.

Tilton, Nan, Todd Tilton, and Gaylen Moore, *Making Miracles: In Vitro Fertilization*. Garden City, NY: Doubleday & Co., Inc., 1985.

Surrogate Motherhood

Andrews, Lori, *New Conceptions*. New York: St. Martin's Press, 1984.

Gelman, David, and Daniel Shapiro, "Infertility: Babies by Contract," *Newsweek*, November 4, 1985, pp. 74–76.

Keane, Noel P., with Dennis Breo, *The Surrogate Mother*. New York: Everest House, 1981.

"Who Keeps 'Baby M'?" *Newsweek*, January 19, 1987, pp. 44–51.

Adoption

Arms, Suzanne, *To Love and Let Go*. New York: Alfred A. Knopf, 1983. (Profiles of birthmothers who have released infants for adoption.)

Bolles, Edmund Blair, *The Penguin Adoption Handbook*. New York: Penguin Books, 1984.

Canape, Charlene, *Adoption: Parenthood Without Pregnancy*. New York: Henry Holt & Co., Inc., 1986.

Gilman, Lois, *The Adoption Resource Book*. New York: Harper and Row Publishers, 1984.

Gilman, Lois, "Adoption: How to Do It on Your Own," *Money*, October 1985, pp. 161–168.

Gradstein, Bonnie, Marc Gradstein, and Robert Glass, M.D., "Private Adoption," *Fertility and Sterility*, 37:4, April 1982, pp. 548–552.

Johnston, Patricia Irwin, *An Adopter's Advocate*. Fort Wayne, IN: Perspectives Press, 1984. (See Resources and Organizations for address.)

Johnston, Patricia Irwin, ed., *Perspectives on a Grafted Tree*. Fort Wayne, IN: Perspectives Press, 1983. (A collection of poetry on adoption.)

Kline, David, "He's Ours . . . He's Really Ours," *McCalls*, March 1984, pp. 56–57.

Krementz, Jill, *How It Feels to Be Adopted*. New York: Knopf, 1982.

Plumez, Jacqueline Hornar, *Successful Adoption*. New York: Harmony Books, 1982.

Artificial Insemination by Donor (AID)

Curie-Cohen, Martin, et al., "Current Practice of Artificial Insemination by Donor in the United States," *New England Journal of Medicine*, March 15, 1979, pp. 585–590.

Menning, Barbara Eck, "Psychological Issues in Artificial Insemination by Donor," *Contemporary Ob/Gyn*, 18:4, October 1981, pp. 155–172.

Noble, Elizabeth, *Having Your Baby by Donor Insemination: The Complete Resource Guide*. Boston: Houghton Mifflin Co., 1987.

Wallis, Claudia, et al., "The New Origins of Life," *Time*, September 10, 1984, pp. 46–53.

Childfree Living

Bombardieri, Merle, *The Baby Decision: How to Make the Most Important Choice of Your Life*. New York: Rawson, Wade Publishers, Inc., 1981. (Order from Merle Bombardieri, 26 Trapelo Rd., Belmont, MA 02178, $9.95 paper, $13.95 hardcover.)

Faux, Marian, *Childless by Choice: Choosing Childlessness in the Eighties*. New York: Doubleday, 1984.

Lindsay, Karen, *Friends as Family*. Boston: Beacon Press, 1981.

Shealy, C. Norman, M.D., and Mary Charlotte Shealy, *To Parent or Not?* Virginia Beach, VA: The Donning Co., 1981.

"Three's a Crowd," *Newsweek*, September 1, 1986, pp. 68–76.

Whelan, Elizabeth M., *A Baby? . . . Maybe*. New York: The Bobbs-Merrill Co., Inc., 1975.

Parenting

Boston Women's Health Book Collective, *Ourselves and Our Children*. New York: Random House, 1978.

Friedland, Ronnie, and Carol Kant, eds., *The Mother Book*. Boston: Houghton Mifflin Co., 1981. (Chapters on foster and adoptive parenting, pregnancy after infertility, miscarriage and stillbirth.)

Hawke, Sharryl, and David Knox, *One Child by Choice*. New York: Prentice Hall Press, 1977.

Kappleman, Murray, M.D., *Raising the Only Child*. New York: New American Library, 1977.

McCauley, Carole, *Pregnancy After 35*. New York: E. P. Dutton, 1976.

Nance, Sherri, *Premature Babies: A Handbook for Parents*. New York: Arbor House, 1982.

Procacci, Joseph, and Mark Kiefaber, *Parent Burnout*. Garden City, NY: Doubleday & Co., Inc., 1983.

Coping and Problem Solving

Barbach, Lonnie, *For Each Other: Sharing Sexual Intimacy*. Garden City, NY: Anchor Press/Doubleday, 1982.

Benson, Herbert, M.D., *The Relaxation Response*. New York: William Morrow & Co., 1975; Avon Books, 1977.

Broderick, Carlfred, *Couples: How to Confront Problems and Maintain Loving Relationships*. New York: Simon and Schuster, 1979.

Hanes, Mari, *Beyond Heartache*. Wheaton, IL: Tyndale House, 1984.

Johnston, Patricia Irwin, *Understanding*. Fort Wayne, IN: Perspectives Press, 1983.

Kushner, Harold, *When Bad Things Happen to Good People*. New York: Schocken Books, 1981.

Linn, Dennis, and Matthew Linn, *Healing Life's Hurts*. Ramsey, NJ: Paulist Press, 1978.

Rubin, Theodore Isaac, *Reconciliations: Inner Peace in an Age of Anxiety*. New York: Viking Press, 1980.

Scarf, Maggie, *Intimate Partners: Patterns in Love and Marriage*. New York: Random House, 1987.

Stearns, Ann Kaiser, *Living Through Personal Crisis*. New York: Ballantine Books, 1985.

Tatlebaum, Judy, *The Courage to Grieve*. New York: Harper and Row, 1980.

Resources and Organizations

Infertility Organizations

RESOLVE, Inc., 5 Water St., Arlington, MA 02174 (617-643-2424). A national, nonprofit organization for infertile individuals and couples and for associated professionals. There are more than 40 chapters throughout the United States. Services include phone counseling, referral to medical and related services, support groups, seminars for the public and for professionals, fact sheets on infertility and alternatives, and an excellent national newsletter.

American Fertility Society, 2131 Magnolia Ave., Suite 201, Birmingham, AL 35256 (205-251-9764). The national membership organization for health professionals with a specialty or interest in infertility. Will provide medical referrals by sending a list of doctors in your area, but will not give recommendations. They publish the monthly journal *Fertility and Sterility* and sponsor excellent seminars for professionals in areas of infertility.

Specialized Organizations

Endometriosis Association, P.O. Box 92187, Milwaukee, WI 53202 (414-962-9031). A self-help organization for women with endometriosis. More than 40 chapters and an excellent newsletter. Services include crisis hotline, support groups, fact sheets, and educational programs.

Compassionate Friends, (national office) P.O. Box 1347, Oak Brook, IL 60521 (312-323-5010). Has chapters throughout the country and provides support and information to couples who have experienced pregnancy loss.

DES Action, 2845 24th St., San Francisco, CA 94110 (415-826-5060). Has a national newsletter and local chapters dealing with DES related issues.

Hysterectomy Educational Resources and Services, 501 Woodbrook Lane, Philadelphia, PA 19119 (215-247-6232). Publishes a newsletter dealing with information about surgery, estrogen replacement therapy, and postsurgical concerns.

American Association of Sex Educators, Counselors, and Therapists, 5010 Wisconsin Ave., N.W., Suite 304, Washington, DC 20016. Publishes booklets on sexual topics. Also gives referrals to local therapists affiliated with the organization.

Adoption Resources

North American Council on Adoptable Children (NACAC), 810 18th St., N.W., Suite 703, Washington, DC 20006 (202-466-7570). Has information on placement of special needs and older children, publishes a newsletter, and has a network of parent support groups.

OURS, Inc., 3307 Highway 100 North, Suite 203, Minneapolis, MN 55442 (612-535-4829). Publishes a newsletter and has a listing of adoption agencies doing international adoptions.

Parents for Private Adoption, P.O. Box 7, Pawlet, VT 05761. Publishes a newsletter and provides information on the subject of legal private adoptions.

Perspectives Press, 905 W. Wildwood Ave., Fort Wayne, IN 46807. A small publishing house dedicated to publications dealing with issues of adoption and infertility. Write to them for a brochure of their books and a current price list.

Index